# You, Me
## and
# Myasthenia Gravis

### Third Edition

by
**Deborah Cavel-Greant**

**Medical Editor**
**Michael W. Nicolle MD, FRCPC, D.Phil.**

# Ku:reh Press

You, Me and Myasthenia Gravis

**Canadian Cataloguing in Publication Data**

Cavel-Greant, Deborah, 1946 -
You, Me and Myasthenia Gravis

Includes bibliographical references

ISBN 0-9693955-2-3

1. Myasthenia gravis -- popular works
 I. Title

Printed in Canada

This book is meant to educate and should not be used as an alternative for professional medical care. Every effort has been made to ensure that the information presented herein is accurate at the time of publication, however there is no guarantee that the information will remain current over time. Consult the appropriate medical professionals for medical advice and treatment.

First Edition – 1988
Second Edition (updated) 1993

# TABLE OF CONTENTS:

Preface:

## ACKNOWLEDGMENTS:

The author wishes to aknowledge the kindness and generosity of the following, whose professional and/or financial contributions helped make this edition possible.

Lidia Cosentino Ph.D. of Bayer Healthcare Canada

Michael Nicolle, MD, FRCPC, D.Phil.

Myasthenia Gravis Association of British Columbia

Valeant Canada Limitée/Limited

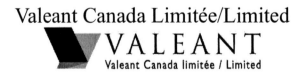

## DEDICATION

This book is dedicated to the memories of my beloved sister, Ruby Cavel O'Connor and my friend Jackie Burch, who both left us in 2005. I'll miss both of them forever.

## MANY THANKS TO:

My family, who are my daily joy; My husband of 40 years, Tony; Our sons, Ian and Zak, and beautiful daughter-in-law Mandy; Dr. Virginia Clark, who is a model physician, and is always there when we need her; Dr. Lidia Cosentino, for her encouragement and extraordinary kindness; Dr. Mike Nicolle, for his meticulous editing; and Mark Carey, for his encouragement and enthusiasm for this project.

To my dear friends Audrey Withers, who was in the right place at the right time and Iris Biteen, without whom I'd never had the courage and persistance to finish this book, and my much-loved friend of many years, Jackie Burch, who I met through the first edition and who slipped away unexpectedly only weeks before this edition was done.

To Judy Bonny, Brenda Kelsey, Bob Langlois, Lynn Waltz and Marika Bates who have cheered me on through this long rewrite.

Also, many thanks to those patients who graciously shared their personal stories with us. I could not have done it without all of you, caring for me, acting as my advocates and providing exactly the help I needed, when I needed it most.

With great affection and gratitude,

*Deborah*

# PREFACE

When faced with the onset of an illness, one of the greatest obstacles to securing a correct diagnosis is a lack of information. This is all too true for myasthenia gravis and related disorders. There is often a long delay before a diagnosis of myasthenia gravis is reached, in part because of the sometimes subtle and often variable weakness which accompanies this disorder. As a physician I have seen hundreds of patients with myasthenia gravis go through frustration, despair and uncertainty, but eventually they find hope and then triumph as treatment is started and the benefits are obtained.

The book you have before you is one of the biggest assets a patient or family member with myasthenia gravis, a congenital myasthenic syndrome or a related disorder of neuromuscular transmission can have. It is much easier to face the difficulties ahead when you understand what is happening, what is being done in terms of investigations, and why therapies are suggested.

Ms. Cavel-Greant has in this volume done an excellent job of providing the information needed to understand myasthenia gravis, its investigation and treatment, as well as the current "state of the art" knowledge of the congenital myasthenic syndromes. This book will serve as an excellent reference for those patients with myasthenia gravis and their loved ones.

It has been over a decade since the 2nd Edition of *You, Me and Myasthenia Gravis* was published, and much has changed. There are new tools available for the diagnosis of myasthenia and congenital myasthenic syndromes, and new treatments available. Although the early stages of treatment are often frustrating, eventually most patients with acquired myasthenia gravis improve and can lead a normal life. With further research the hope is that a treatment will be found which will benefit all MG patients, and eventually that more long lasting forms of therapy, approaching the holy grail of a "cure", will be found.

Michael Nicolle, MD, FRCPC, D. Phil.

# 1

# MYASTHENIA

## A BRIEF BIOLOGY

Myasthenia gravis (MG) is a chronic neuromuscular[1] disease which affects the strength and stamina of voluntary muscles[2]. The symptoms of MG result from an immune system attack on structures in the neuromuscular junction (NMJ), the junction between a nerve fiber and the muscle it supplies.

A second very rare type of myasthenia, the congenital myasthenic syndrome[3] (CMS), is caused by a genetic mutation[4] which can be passed from parent to child. The symptoms of the congenital myasthenias result from changes in function at the NMJ. These changes vary depending on the genetic mutation.

This book seeks to explain how myasthenia, both autoimmune/acquired, and congenital, affects the body. It explains MG treatments and how they work, and it shares the experiences of both physicians and patients. We know more about myasthenia now than ever before. But to understand this knowledge we need to learn about nerves, muscles and the immune system. In this chapter we'll examine how nerves and muscles work together to produce movement, and how the neuromuscular junction (where the problem is in MG) works. We'll see how the immune system tells the difference between self and non-self, how it protects us from attack by

---

1  Neuromuscular: Involving both the nerves and muscles.
2  Voluntary muscles: Muscles which we exercise conscious control over, such as the muscles of the legs and jaw.
3  Syndrome: A group of signs and symptoms that occur together and are typical of a particular disease or disorder.
4  Genetic mutation: An error in one of the genes encoding one or more proteins.

outside invaders, and finally how errors made by the immune system produce autoimmune diseases like MG. This knowledge will enable us to understand the information in later chapters, give us greater insight into what is happening in the body, and enable us to be better members of our own health care team.

## TRANSLATING INTENTION INTO ACTION

When we reach out to pick up a glass of water we never think of the intricate chemical and electrical dance the *idea* of movement sets off. The intention to pick up the glass forms in the brain, but the command to pick up the glass races from the brain and down the spinal cord in the form of an electrical pulse called an *action potential*.

The action potential speeds from the spinal cord to the end of the motor nerves[5] where it is transformed into a chemical signal, crosses the synapse[6], and on the other side, is transformed back into an action potential, which initiates muscle movement. The glass is then picked up.

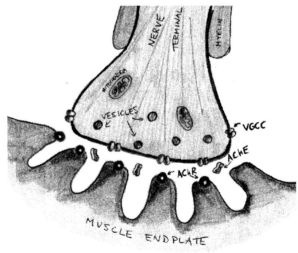

**The motor nerve terminal, containing ACh vesicles and voltage-gated calcium channels, the synapse and muscle endplate. (Drawing courtesy M. Nicolle MD)**

---

5  Motor nerves: Nerves which carry signals to muscle, and are involved in movement.
6  Synapse: a tiny gap that physically separates neurons.

Motor nerves end in bulb-like structures called axon (or nerve) terminals. Nerve terminals make contact with muscle fibers at a region called the *endplate*. The nerve terminal contains *vesicles*[7], which store and release the neurotransmitter[8] acetylcholine (ACh).

Cells are enclosed in a thin wrapper called a membrane. There is an electrical gradient across this membrane. The outside of the membrane has a more positive charge than the inside. When an action potential arrives at the nerve ending it causes an instant reversal of this polarity, which opens calcium channels on the nerve terminal. Calcium ions flowing into the nerve terminal causes acetylcholine (ACh) vesicles to open and release ACh into the NMJ.

## THE PRODUCTION OF ACETYLCHOLINE

Acetylcholine (ACh) is produced by the binding of choline to acetate. Cofactor A, carrying acetate, sticks to the enzyme choline acetyltransferase. The acetate and choline molecules then stick together, producing ACh. After the reaction is complete, the cofactor A molecule is released. The ACh is then packaged and stored in vesicles at the nerve terminal, ready to be released when an action potential arrives.

## ENDPLATE POTENTIALS

When an *action potential* arrives at the nerve terminal, it triggers the release of ACh from 100 - 300 vesicles. Each vesicle contains one *quantum* (10,000 molecules) of ACh. This release of ACh produces an endplate potential (EPP) and starts the process of muscle movement by depolarizing the membrane around it and producing an action potential in the muscle fiber.

## MEPPs

The arrival of an action potential triggers results in muscle movement, but vesicles also leak ACh at a rate of about one per second. This slow leak of ACh cause what are called miniature endplate potentials (MEPPs). MEPPs don't cause enough depolarization of the muscle membrane to trigger movement. There's no clear understanding of the significance of this release of small quantities of ACh and the resulting MEPPs, but we know they play a

---

7   Vesicle: A small bubble filled with chemical.
8   Neurotransmitter: Any chemical that results in the movement of a nerve signal across a synapse.

role in the health of the muscle. They may help maintain muscle tone, as youngsters with less than a normal release of MEPPs have less muscle tone than normal.

## THE NEUROMUSCULAR JUNCTION

Because this system works on electrical principals and the *charge* (action potential) is passed along by the release of ACh, it's important that the "live wires" (so to speak) are not in contact. The nerve terminal and the muscle membrane do not touch. There is a small gap between them, called a *synapse* or *synaptic cleft*. The nerve terminal, the synapse and the muscle membrane are collectively referred to as the *neuromuscular junction (NMJ)*.

### AGRIN, MuSK AND RAPSYN

The synaptic cleft contains a substance called the *basal lamina* which separates the nerve and muscle cell membranes. The basal lamina also plays a vital role in rebuilding the synapse after an injury. Basal lamina contains a protein called *agrin*. When agrin is added to a lab culture containing muscle cells AChRs gather and grow in the muscle membrane.

Motor nerves secrete agrin and deposit it in the basal lamina at the site of the developing NMJ. Agrin acts at its receptor on the surface of the muscle, helping assemble and stabilize acetylcholine receptors (AChRs). In lab mice which have been genetically altered to lack agrin, AChRs do not gather under the axon terminal and NMJs do not form.

The key components of the agrin receptor are a receptor called muscle specific kinase *(MuSK)* and the protein it activates, *rapsyn*. MuSK and rapsyn attract immature AChRs to the area beneath the nerve terminal, causing them to cluster at the endplate and mature into fully functional AChRs. The basal lamina, agrin, MuSK and rapsyn are vital components in the constant regeneration of AChRs. Their function is affected in seronegative MG and some forms of congenital myasthenic syndrome, reducing the number of AChRs which form and mature at the neuromuscular junction.

### ACETYLCHOLINESTERASE

The synaptic cleft also contains the enzyme[9] acetylcholinesterase (AChE). When an action potential arrives and ACh floods the synaptic

---

9   Enzyme: A protein that causes or speeds up reactions in living matter.

cleft it immediately comes into contact with AChE. Acetylcholinesterase begins to break ACh down as soon as the two come into contact. Some ACh is neutralized before it has a chance to bind to ACh receptor sites, but enough reaches and binds to ACh receptor sites to create an *endplate potential* (EPP). Endplate potentials must last for precisely the right amount of time, and generate exactly the right amount of current, for depolarization of the muscle fiber to occur. Thus, after binding briefly to the receptor, ACh is dislodged and either floats out of the NMJ or is broken down by AChE.

## Ion Channels

Ion channels are gateways (or pores) through cell membranes. They allow molecules of potassium, calcium, sodium or chloride to pass in and out of cells. Each type of ion channel responds to a specific signal. The signal may be a change in voltage (like an action potential), a change in temperature, or a chemical stimulus, like a molecule of ACh.

When the appropriate signal arrives the ion channel opens. Most ion channels allow only one type of ion; sodium, potassium, calcium or chloride to pass through. Opposites attract; positively-charged ions move toward a negative charge and vice versa. A membrane may contain many thousands of ion channels. The surge of ions across the membrane generates tiny electrical currents that, in the skeletal muscle cell, begins the process of muscle contraction.

Ion channels are made up of sub-units assembled in groups of four, five or six, depending on the function of the channel. There are six types of voltage-gated calcium channels (VGCC). They are identified by the letters L, N, R, P, Q and T. The calcium channels on the axon terminal are P and Q types. P and Q calcium channels are made up of subunits alpha1, alpha2, beta, gamma, and delta.

The ion channel is essentially a pore through the membrane which opens and closes in response to the appropriate signal. When the signal arrives and binds to the one subunit which serves as the receptor, the entire ion channel opens. Ions of the proper shape or charge can then flow through. When the signaling period expires, the tube snaps closed and molecules stop flowing.

## THE ACETYLCHOLINE RECEPTOR

The acetylcholine receptor (AChR) spans the muscle cell membrane. The adult AChR is made up of five subunits; two alpha units, one beta unit, one epsilon unit, and one delta unit. Each subunit is encoded[10] by a separate gene. The five subunits are arranged in a tubular shape around a ligand-gated[11] ion channel, like the staves in a barrel.

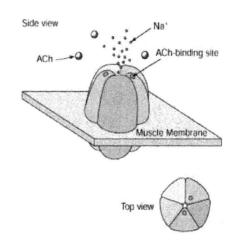

**AChR spanning the muscle membrane, and as seen from above. (Courtesy M. Nicolle MD)**

The two alpha units each have binding sites for ACh. When two ACh molecules bind to the alpha units the complex changes shape and the ion channel opens. The channel remains open for about one millisecond and then snaps closed. The ACh molecules are then released from the receptors, fall into the synapse and are broken down by AChE. The AChR then reverts to the closed state.

Acetylcholine is the key that opens the ion channel. When ACh binds to the receptor site it causes depolarization of the muscle membrane. If the amount of depolarization is enough an action potential is generated in the muscle membrane. Sodium channels open, sodium ions flow into the muscle cell which triggers the release of calcium ions inside the cell. The release of calcium ions then causes muscle contraction or movement.

## ACH RECEPTOR TYPES

ACh receptors are constantly being replaced. There are two types of AChRs. The majority are of the so-called stable type. At least 50% of these are replaced every 12 - 13 days. The second type of receptors

---

10 Encode: To specify the genetic code for.
11 Ligand-gated: Permitting or blocking passage through a cell membrane in response to a chemical stimulus.

(called RTOs for *rapid turnover*) are replaced much more quickly. Fifty percent of them break down and are replaced on a daily basis. Although RTOs make up only 20 - 30% of the total number of receptor sites they account for almost 70% of the overall turnover. Not all RTOs break down this quickly, six to ten percent stabilize and become the longer-lived type.

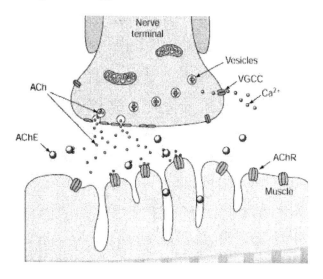

**The neuromuscular junction, showing the AChRs in place on the muscle membrane. (Drawing courtesy M. Nicolle MD)**

The production of two types of AChRs makes sense. If all receptors were of the stable type it would take far longer for the body to recover from an agent that blocked or interrupted neuromuscular transmission. If all receptors were RTOs the body would have to expend far more resources constantly making their replacements. A two-tiered system thus both conserves and protects neuromuscular function.

Surprisingly, normal neuromuscular transmission requires that only 25 - 30% of the total number of AChRs be functional at any one time. Patients may have a 50 - 60% reduction of AChRs and still show no clinical signs of inadequate neuromuscular transmission.

## THE IMMUNE SYSTEM AND MG

The immune system is a network designed to protect the body from invasion by bacteria, viruses, molds, parasites or any type of foreign substance. The organs of the immune system are located throughout the body. They are called lymphoid organs because they produce, regulate and, in some cases, deliver lymphocytes; white blood cells that are the main components of the immune system.

### SELF AND NON-SELF

The very foundation of the immune system is its ability to distinguish *self* from *non-self*. Immune cells live in a state known as *self-tolerance,* because every cell in a person's body carries a unique *self-marker*. These self-markers (called *epitopes*) protrude from the surfaces of every cell. Every  epitope has a unique shape which functions like a key. The immune system is constantly checking cells it meets for epitopes. It recognizes its own epitope as the *self-marker*. In a healthy body the immune system does not attack organs or tissues with the self-marker.

The immune system recognizes *non-self* tissues by the *foreign* shape of its protruding epitopes. The immune system has the ability to recognize unlimited numbers of different non-self molecules and can produce antibodies to counteract each of them.

### ANTIGENS

The parts of proteins which trigger an immune response are known as antigens. Antigens are found on viruses, bacteria, molds, and body cells or tissues, which is why transplanted organs such as a kidney or heart trigger a *rejection* response. The rejection response is the immune system attacking tissues it has identified as non-self.

### HUMAN LEUKOCYTE ANTIGENS

Human leukocyte antigens (HLA) are proteins found in most cell membranes in the body. There are high concentrations of HLAs on the surface of white blood cells. The immune system also uses HLA antigens to tell self from non-self. There are many different HLA proteins. Individuals have only a small, relatively unique set inherited from their parents. Two unrelated people rarely have the same HLA make-up.

We inherit one-half of our HLA antigens from our parents. One quarter of our antigens matches our mother's antigens, and one-quarter matches our father's antigens. The remaining 50% of our antigens are drawn from the genetic pool of previous ancestors. This mix becomes crucial when a person needs a tissue graft or organ transplant when it is vital that the patient's antigens match the donor's antigens. An HLA incompatibility may make an organ from a patient's brother or sister unsuitable for transplant.

## IMMUNE SYSTEM CELLS

Immune cells develop in the bone marrow from *stem cells*[12]. Some stem cells develop into white blood cells known as phagocytes or macrophages. Phagocytes destroy invaders by engulfing and digesting them. A small number of phagocytes become specialized inflammatory cells. Other stem cells develop into white blood cells called *lymphocytes*. The two major kinds of lymphocytes are *B cells* and *T cells*. *B cells* produce substances known as antibodies. When a B cell meets its triggering antigen it begins to mature into large numbers of plasma cells. These plasma cells then begin producing quantities of their specific antibody.

*T cells* play two roles in the immune system. They first develop in the bone marrow, along with the B cells, but those destined to become T cells leave the bone marrow and migrate to the *thymus*, where they learn to recognize self and non-self antigens. This is the reason they are called thymus-dependent lymphocyte or *T cells*.

*Helper T cells* activate other immune cells including B cells and other T cells. *Suppressor T cells* turn off or suppress immune activity when the invader has been killed and the clean-up is over. *Cytotoxic T cells* help rid the body of cells that have been infected by viruses as well as cells that have been affected by cancer. Cytotoxic T cells are also responsible for the rejection of tissue and organ transplants.

## THE THYMUS

The *thymus* is a gland located just behind the breastbone and in front of the heart. It teaches the T cells to ignore self antigens and attack foreign antigens. Some T cells help regulate the immune system, while others act as defenders against viral infection and cancerous tissues.

---

12 Stem cell: The most primitive cell in the bone marrow from which all the various types of blood cells are derived.

## ANTIBODIES

Antibodies consist of two identical heavy chains and two identical light chains which fit together to form a Y. The stem of the Y is identical in all antibodies of the same kind and is called the *constant region*. It links the antibody to the rest of the body's defense system. The sections that form the tips of the Y are called the *variable region*. The tips are unique to each type of antibody. They fit onto the epitopes of only one antigen like a key fits into its lock. When an antibody finds its matching antigen it binds to it.

## IMMUNOGLOBULINS

B cells make antibodies, also called *immunoglobulins*. There are nine types of human immunoglobulin; four kinds of IgG and two kinds of IgA, plus IgM, IgE and IgD. IgG, the major immunoglobulin in the blood, is also able to enter tissue where it coats microorganisms, helping other cells in the immune system dispose of them more quickly. IgD is found in the membrane of B cells, where it helps regulate the cell's activation. IgE gives protection against parasites, but also causes allergic reactions.

## THE COMPLEMENT SYSTEM

The *complement* system is made up of a series of proteins that complement the work of antibodies. There are 18 complement proteins (CPs), each with a different job. Complement Proteins circulate in the blood in an inactive form, activating only when needed to fight infection.

The complement system protects the body against infection in several ways. It produces large numbers of activated CPs that bind to the surface of bacterial and viral invaders. These CPs attract macrophages (phagocytes) to the site of complement activation and switch them on once they have arrived. The macrophages respond to the presence of CP on the surface of the invading cells by surrounding and devouring the invader cells. Lastly, a *complement cascade* is activated when complement protein encounters and recognizes an antibody bound to an antigen. These complement proteins assemble a cylinder that punctures the membrane of the cell and helps kill it.

## AUTOIMMUNE DISEASE

Sometimes the immune system's ability to distinguish between self and non-self breaks down, and the immune system produces antibodies and T cells targeted against the body's own cells and organs Antibodies against the self are called *auto*-antibodies. Auto-antibodies contribute to many diseases. Organs and tissues commonly affected by autoimmune disorders include red blood cells, blood vessels, connective tissues, endocrine glands, muscles, joints and skin. For instance, T cells that attack cells in the pancreas contribute to some forms of diabetes, while over 90% of people with the autoimmune disease *Lupus* have *antinuclear antibodies.* Antinuclear antibodies attack the nucleus of cells and tissues. Other autoimmune disorders include rheumatoid arthritis, Graves' disease, chronic thyroiditis (Hashimoto's disease), multiple sclerosis, pernicious anemia and myasthenia gravis.

## ANTIBODIES AND MG

Antibodies to acetylcholine receptor (AChR) are found in approximately 85% of MG patients. Myasthenia gravis is referred to as a *B cell mediated* disease, because B cell auto-antibodies attack the alpha subunit of the AChR. In most cases antibodies are directed against the *main immunogenic region* (MIR)[13] on the alpha subunit. AChR antibodies can cause problems in three ways; they can bind to the AChR and block access by ACh, without damaging the receptor; they can bind to AChRs and damage them, so that the AChRs break down and are absorbed into the muscle; and they can bind complement and damage the muscle endplate. As the number of receptors decrease the NMJ becomes less responsive to ACh. There is reduced transmission of the nerve signal, resulting in muscle weakness.

The role of the thymus in MG cannot be overlooked. T cells, activated in the thymus, do not attack the NMJ directly, but play a role in MG autoimmunity. T cells stimulate AChR-reactive B cells, which results in their transformation into the plasma cells which produce AChR antibodies. Abnormalities of the thymus are common in MG patients.

About 85% of MG patients with generalized weakness have measurable anti-AChR antibodies, but the remaining 15% do not. Patients who do not have identifiable antibodies against the AChR have what is called *Seronegative* [14] MG.

13 MIR: Relating to or producing an immune response.
14 Seronegative: No identifiable antibodies.

## MuSK Antibody and Rapsyn

During development the motor nerve terminal secretes the protein *agrin*, which "wakes up" immature AChRs randomly scattered in the muscle membrane. MuSK and a protein called *rapsyn* then work together to assemble and mature the AChRs. Muscle specific kinase (MuSK) is an enzyme essential to the formation of AChRs during the development of the neuromuscular junction. Studies of MG patients in the seronegative group have revealed that a recently discovered *MuSK* antibody is present in 30 - 50% of patients in this group, suggesting a different mechanism for MG in these patients.

MuSK and rapsyn are vital components in the constant regeneration of AChRs. Some types of the congenital myasthenic syndromes are caused by mutations which affect the production or function of rapsyn.

## There's Hope for Tomorrow!

Knowledge of the immune system and the neuromuscular junction have greatly expanded in the past 15 years. This gives us hope that MG will soon be a disorder which can be quickly brought under control by treatments which suppress the inappropriate autoimmune response while leaving the rest of the immune system intact and functioning normally.

# 2
# THE SYMPTOMS
# OF MYASTHENIA GRAVIS

The symptoms of myasthenia gravis (MG) are the result of an immune system attack on the acetylcholine receptors (AChR) at the neuromuscular junction (NMJ). The muscle groups affected can vary from person to person. Symptoms and their intensity can change daily.

## WHAT ARE THE SYMPTOMS OF MG?

Patients in the early stages of MG often report that they tire rapidly and that it takes longer for them to recover from fatigue than it once did. However, because fatigue is a symptom of many disorders and is experienced by perfectly healthy people at times of physical or emotional stress it is not by itself any real help diagnostically.

Symptoms more specific to MG are related to the inability of affected muscles to contract repeatedly or maintain efficient contraction. Although any skeletal muscle can be affected, MG weakness usually begins in eye or facial muscles or in muscles close to the body (shoulders, hips, upper arms and legs), rather than in hands or feet. The weakness is usually the same on both sides of the body. It usually grows worse with use and patients are often weakest at the end of the day.

The eyes themselves are not affected by MG, but the muscles which control the movement of the eyes and eyelids (ocular muscles) often are. When ocular muscles are affected the eyelids may droop, or it may become hard for the patient to fully open (or close) one or both eyes. It may be difficult for the patient to look to the sides or up and down. An imbalance in the strength of the muscles that coordinate eye movement may cause blurred or double vision. Double vision may come in brief episodes or it may be constant.

If the facial muscles are affected the face may become mask-like or expressionless. The smile may be flat or the patient may be unable to smile at all. This mask-like expression and inability to smile has sometimes led to a diagnosis of depression. Weakness of the tongue, jaw, throat and lips can lead to slurred speech and dropped syllables. The voice may become nasal or weak. Some patients are  unable to speak during periods of weakness.

Weakness may make it difficult for the myasthenic to chew foods like steak or swallow dry foods like potato. Food may become lodged at the back of the throat. Liquids may come back up through the nose. The patient may choke on fluids, including their own saliva. If the muscles at the back of the throat are weak the gag reflex may be lost. The jaw muscles may become too weak to hold the jaw closed, leaving the mouth hanging open. When sitting the patient may hold the jaw closed by propping the chin in the hand.

Though MG is described as painless, patients can experience headaches, neck and back pain caused by the strain of supporting the head with weak neck and upper back muscles. Weakness can complicate the performance of the most basic activities of life. Weakness of hands, arms and shoulder muscles may make it difficult to comb the hair, open doors or jars, or dress oneself. If the hip girdle and leg muscles are weak, walking, climbing stairs and getting in and out of cars become a challenge. Patients may fall and be unable to get up, may need help to stand from a chair or get out of bed or the bathtub. Sitting in an armless chair can be an issue if trunk muscles are weak.

The diaphragm is the main muscle we use to breathe. It acts like a bellows, expanding and contracting the chest with each breath, moving air in and out of the lungs. Weakness of the diaphragm and rib cage muscles can affect the patient's ability to breathe adequately. Patients may experience shortness of breath when lying flat or bending over. Weak muscles at the back of the throat may allow collapse of the upper airway. At one time *myasthenic crisis,* due to weakness or exhaustion of the diaphragm and chest muscles, was common. Crisis is now rare, due to better diagnosis and management.

## CO-EXISTING DISORDERS

Other autoimmune diseases occur more often in patients with MG than in the general population. The fact that autoimmune diseases tend to cluster in a patient, or family, suggests that autoimmunity itself stems from a basic inability of the immune system to recognize self versus non-self. Some autoimmune diseases that occur more often in MG patients are thyroid disease, pernicious anemia (vitamin B-12 deficiency), rheumatoid arthritis and lupus.

Tachycardia (a rapid heart rate) or exophthalmos[15] point to the possibility of an overactive thyroid gland, which is present in 10 - 15% of patients with MG. An equal number of MG patients have hypothyroidism - an under active thyroid. These patients may experience muscle weakness, lethargy, intolerance to cold, constipation and a slower than normal heart rate. It's important to have annual thyroid tests because if an MG patient has thyroid gland abnormalities their weakness may not improve until thyroid activity is normalized.

## SLEEP APNEA IN MG

Many MG patients complain that they suffer from poor quality of sleep as well as memory and concentration difficulties. These problems are especially apparent during exacerbations[16] of weakness.

Several studies have described sleep apnea[17] and hypopnea[18] in patients with MG. Apnea and hypopnea usually occur during periods of dreaming (called rapid eye movement or REM sleep). In the general population, older people (especially men) and those who are obese are more likely to develop sleep apnea. In MG patients physical inactivity and treatment with prednisone appear to further contribute to the development of sleep apnea.

In a study of sleep apnea in 100 randomly chosen MG patients authored by Michael Nicolle et. al. (in press) the overall prevalence of sleep apnea was at least 36%, compared to the expected prevalence of 5% in the general population.

Sleep apnea is not caused by the medications used to treat MG, or by antibodies to muscle AChRs. AChRs in the brain are structurally different from skeletal AChRs and are not affected.

Although sleep apnea is not directly associated with the severity of a patient's MG, it becomes less of a problem as MG symptoms improve, so there must be a link. The question becomes - what is it?

It's thought that the critical factors may be total lung capacity as well as weakness of the diaphragm. Oxygen levels drop in everyone

---

15  Exophthalmos: Abnormal protrusion of the eyeball.
16  Exacerbation: A period of time when symptoms of a disease become more severe.
17  Sleep apnea: A temporary pause in breathing during sleep.
18  Hypopnea: Abnormally slow or shallow respiration.

during REM sleep. During REM sleep MG patients who have weakness of pharyngeal and/or respiratory muscles are more likely to have sleep apnea. The lower oxygen saturation and disturbed sleep during these periods then contribute to poor memory and other cognitive problems.

In another study, 19 middle-aged patients with MG and 10 controls of the same age, sex and education underwent overnight testing, to see whether memory impairment in MG is related to sleep apnea or is caused by central nervous system involvement. Researchers observed that 60% of the myasthenics experienced sleep apnea and hypopnea with lowered oxygen levels. These myasthenics had decreased memory function. Compared to MG patients without sleep apnea, myasthenics with sleep apnea had impaired memory.

Patients with MG can suffer from respiratory failure during sleep despite normal daytime respiratory function. The normal reduction in muscle tone which occurs during sleep may be life-threatening in a patient with impaired muscle strength. Symptoms may include snoring which pauses and then resumes, pauses in breathing during sleep, an inability to breathe unless propped upright, blueness or greyness of the lips and/or nail beds, restless sleep and insomnia. Daytime symptoms of apnea can include weakness and/or fatigue which does not respond to treatment, morning headaches, excessive daytime sleepiness, irritability and depression. Other symptoms of apnea include polycythemia[19], hypertension and signs of heart failure. Those with sleep apnea also have an increased risk of stroke.

Any MG patient with symptoms of sleep apnea, hypopnea or hypoventilation[20] should be referred to a sleep specialist for a *sleep study*. The patient's blood pressure, breathing rate, heart rate, muscle activity, eye movements and brain waves are recorded during a night of sleep to determine if the sleep and breathing patterns are normal.

Treatment options for apnea include noninvasive ventilation such as the continuous positive airway pressure (C-PAP) and bi-level positive airway pressure (Bi-PAP) machines. Treatment for apnea improves the quality of life for most patients, lessens the risk of developing other lung or heart disease, and decreases the risk of stroke.

---

19 Polycythemia: An abnormally high red blood cell count.
20 Hypoventilation: Deficient ventilation of the lungs that results in reduction in the oxygen content or increase in the carbon dioxide content of the blood or both.

It's reassuring to know that the memory lapses and other cognitive dysfunctions reported by patients are almost certainly due to sleep disturbances and the slightly lower oxygen levels which occur during dreaming periods, rather than by brain damage or impairment. It is important that patients who have symptoms of sleep apnea speak to the physician because there is safe, effective treatment available which will improve the quality of life.

## VARIABILITY OF SYMPTOMS

Few myasthenics have the entire range of possible symptoms. In addition, symptoms may vary in intensity daily or even hourly. This variability of symptoms can contribute to the difficulty of getting a diagnosis. It's also one of the most frustrating aspects of the disease. Any type of stress, physical or mental, tends to make the symptoms of MG worse. Injury, surgery and pain are physical stresses that may cause MG to flare temporarily. Fever in particular is a major cause of exacerbations in MG patients. Increased weakness may linger months after an infection has subsided. This has always been something of a puzzle, but research has shed new light on why the myasthenic continues to produce antibodies long after they should have stopped.

In a person with a normally functioning immune system *suppressor cells* stop the production of antibodies once an infection is overcome. But when blood taken from an MG patient is put into a culture of suppressor cells (taken from unaffected individuals) immune cells from the MG blood block the ability of the suppressor cells to turn off antibody production. This means that the immune system of an MG patient probably continues vigorous antibody production longer than it should, producing antibodies which attack the NMJ and prolong weakness.

Living with MG is a daily challenge which calls on one's deepest reserves of strength. Thankfully, with the advances in treatment it should not be the life-threatening challenge it once was.

## NOTES:

# 3

# HOW IS MG DIAGNOSED?

The diagnosis of myasthenia gravis (MG) continues to be a medical challenge. It is not unusual to find myasthenics who have experienced symptoms for months, or even years, before a definitive diagnosis was reached.

When a patient develops the classic symptoms of drooping eyelids, double vision and easily observable muscular weakness, the diagnosis is usually straight-forward. But since MG occurs in only one person of 7,000 - 10,000 many family physicians may never encounter a patient, and may not recognize the symptoms. It is not unusual for a patient to see several physicians during their quest for a diagnosis. Patients whose symptoms do not include ocular involvement, or who experience a slow or fluctuating onset, can face a diagnostic labyrinth.

In 1990 the prevalence of diagnosed MG in the USA was estimated at 7.5 - 12.5 cases per 100,000 persons. More recently the prevalence was estimated at 14 cases per 100,000. This rise in case numbers does not indicate that MG is increasing, but that physicians are getting better at diagnosing it, which is *very* encouraging. However, many authorities in the field still feel that MG is under diagnosed and that the prevalence is still probably higher than reported. This is partially because MG can be difficult to diagnose in early or mild cases. But it can also be due to the fact that there are still physicians who are relatively unaware of the disease. Since tiredness or fatigability is a common complaint the undiagnosed myasthenic can be seen by these physicians as "just a complainer".

On the other hand, patients may experience symptoms for years before they even consult a physician. There may be a remarkable degree of adaption to slow-onset weakness that even the patient is unaware of. Adaptation to some aspects of the disability may be so successful that the patient may deny that they have a problem.

## THE TYPICAL PATIENT IS CHANGING

The face of MG is also changing. The typical MG patient of 20 years ago may not be today's typical patient. In the past, women were more frequently affected with MG than men. In women the most common age for onset has always been in the second and third decades. In men onset was most often during the seventh and eighth decades. As the population ages the average age at onset has increased. Men are now more often affected than women with the age of onset usually after 50.

This change in the typical presentation of MG may make it more difficult for some patients to get a diagnosis. However, overall, the awareness of MG seems higher than it was in 1988, when the first edition of this book was published. Thankfully the speed with which most patients are diagnosed seems to have accelerated.

The most important factor in the diagnostic process is the skill of the physician who interviews the patient. The physician must take a thorough medical history and *listen carefully* to the patient's observations regarding his own condition. These are essential first steps. The interview should then be followed by a general physical exam, followed by a neurological exam. If at this point the physician suspects MG he will usually arrange for a number of tests to be done.

## DIAGNOSTIC TESTS FOR MG

There is no single diagnostic test that will catch every case of MG, though some of the newer ones come close.

## LABORATORY STUDIES

The following three tests check for antibodies in the blood, so a blood sample will be drawn, and sent to a special diagnostic lab.

### ANTI-ACETYLCHOLINE RECEPTOR ANTIBODY TEST

A positive anti-acetylcholine receptor (anti-AChR) antibody test is viewed as proof of MG since approximately 85% of myasthenics with generalized MG, and 50% of those with ocular MG, have anti-AChR antibodies. False positives are rare, but do occur occasionally in cases of thymoma without MG and in a small number of otherwise healthy people over 70 years of age.

## MUSCLE SPECIFIC KINASE ANTIBODY TEST

If the anti-AChR antibody test is negative a Muscle Specific Kinase (*MuSK* positive) antibody test can be ordered. This test has become available only recently, since the MuSK positive antibody was only discovered in 2001. MuSK positive MG develops when a person develops antibodies to the MuSK receptors at the NMJ. (See Chapter Four) MuSK positive MG is found in about seven percent of MG patients.

## SERONEGATIVE MG

MG patients who do not have identifiable antibodies now comprise only 7 - 8% of patients. These patients are called s*eronegative*.

## IMAGING TESTS

Between 75 - 80% of all MG patients with anti-AChR antibodies have abnormalities of the thymus. Thymoma (tumor of the thymus) occurs eventually in about 15% of MG patients. Every MG patient with anti-AChR antibodies should be checked for thymoma. Several imaging tests are used to locate a thymoma and determine its boundaries. Most thymomas are benign. About 60% of anti-AChR antibody positive patients have thymic hyperplasia (an abnormal multiplication of thymus cells). Another 35% have an involuted thymus (one which has shrunk and degenerated), although this is not abnormal in an adult. Since thymectomy[21] is a frequently used form of treatment for anti-AChR antibody positive MG it is important to know if a patient has thymus involvement.

## COMPUTED TOMOGRAPHY (CT OR CAT SCAN)

The CT scan is a sophisticated X-ray machine that produces detailed cross-sectional images of the body. Instead of taking one X-ray, a CT scanner takes dozens of pictures as it rotates around the patient. A computer then turns these pictures into sectional images, like slices of the body, which are very detailed. A CT scan should be done in every patient who has anti-AChR antibodies.

---

21 Thymectomy: The surgical removal of the thymus gland.

A CT scan can provide precise information about the size, shape, and position of a thymoma, and can help guide decisions about surgical and therapeutic options.

## Nerve Conduction Studies

Electrodiagnostic tests for myasthenia gravis generally involve three components; nerve conduction studies, electromyography and specific tests of neuromuscular transmission.

Nerve conduction studies involve administering small electrical shocks to motor nerves which supply muscles, or to sensory nerves on the skin, to test their function. These studies are most often normal in a patient with myasthenia gravis and are done to exclude other disease processes which may produce similar symptoms. Nevertheless they should be done before specific tests of neuromuscular transmission as it becomes very difficult to interpret some of the testing (SFEMG in particular) unless results of the nerve conduction studies are known.

### Electromyography

The second component is electromyography (EMG), in which a small needle is inserted in the muscle tissue to look for evidence of nerve problems supplying that muscle, or of diseases affecting the muscle itself. Again, these studies are often normal in patients with myasthenia gravis, although subtle abnormalities can be detected by experienced examiners. They are usually done to look for evidence of a muscle disease which could produce similar symptoms to MG. However, there are some cases in which patients with MG may have abnormalities on EMG studies, thought to be because of "functional denervation" in which the defect in neuromuscular transmission is so severe that the muscle tissue becomes irritable, seen on needle EMG as an increase in "spontaneous activity".

### Repetitive Nerve Stimulation

The specific electrodiagnostic tests for MG include repetitive nerve stimulation (RNS) and single fibre EMG. In repetitive nerve stimulation, a nerve supplying a muscle is stimulated repeatedly (often three times per second for anywhere between four and 10 stimuli), looking for a gradual reduction in the size of the measured response, or *decrement*. Other diseases can produce mild degrees of decrement on RNS studies, but if a very significant degree of decrement is seen (over 20%) it is almost always due to myasthenia gravis. RNS can be normal in milder cases of myasthenia, and is often normal in patients with ocular MG. However, when abnormal it is more specific (less likely to be positive in other diseases) for the diagnosis of myasthenia gravis.

## SINGLE FIBRE ELECTROMYOGRAPHY

The most sensitive diagnostic test for problems with neuromuscular transmission (i.e. myasthenia) is single fibre electromyography (SFEMG). This is the test most likely to be abnormal in patients with MG. In this test a small needle is inserted into muscle tissue, in order to be able to measure the electrical response from two small muscle fibres being supplied by the same nerve. If things work normally the variation in arrival times of the electrical signal from these two muscle fibres is more or less constant. If there is a problem at one or more of the neuromuscular junctions supplying these muscle fibres, the arrival times may vary significantly (causing what is called *jitter*) or sometimes the response from one of the muscle fibres doesn't occur at all (blocking).

Almost any muscle in the body can be tested with SFEMG, but muscles commonly tested include those around the eye, on the forehead or on the back of the forearm.

Although highly sensitive, the main problem with SFEMG is that the test can be abnormal for many other reasons other than myasthenia, including a number of other nerve or muscle diseases which can produce similar symptoms.

## HOW ELECTRODIAGNOSTIC TESTS ARE DONE

Electrodiagnostic tests are done in a hospital, clinic or doctor's office. CNS and RNS studies and the EMG are often done at the same appointment. The patient lies on a table or bed, and is made comfortable. While these tests can be somewhat painful they are so for only a few seconds at a time. The needles used are extremely fine, about the size of a human hair, and the electrical pulses are tiny and last for only a fraction of a second. The muscle may jump a bit with the electrical pulse. Patients who have ever used a "TENS" muscle stimulating unit at the physiotherapists or gym will be familiar with the sensation of CNS, RNS or EMG.

## PREPARING FOR ELECTRODIAGNOSTIC TESTS

The patient may eat and drink as usual before the test. They should not smoke for at least three hours before the test. The examiner should be made aware if the patient is (1) taking muscle relaxants or an anticholinesterase since these can interfere with test results; (2) has a bleeding problem or takes medications that thin the blood (such as aspirin, warfarin or heparin); (3) has a pacemaker or defibrillator.

## ELECTROMYOGRAPHY PROCEDURE

EMG testing requires two electrodes: a reference electrode; which may be either a metal disc which is placed on the skin, or a fine needle which is inserted just under the skin; and a recording electrode, which is a fine needle that is inserted into the muscle that is being tested. Once the electrodes are in place, the electrical activity in the muscle is recorded while the muscle is at rest. The examiner will ask the patient to contract the muscle with gradually increasing force while the electrical activity in the muscle is recorded. The recording electrode may be repositioned a number of times to record the electrical activity in different areas of the muscle or in different muscles. Electrical activity in the muscle is displayed on a monitor as a line. The activity also produces sound waves which can be heard on a loudspeaker. When a muscle is contracted it sounds like a machine gun. An EMG may take from 45 minutes to two hours.

## THE EDROPHONIUM OR TENSILON® TEST

In MG, the number of acetylcholine receptor sites at the NMJ is reduced. This results in a reduction of response to acetylcholine (ACh). When ACh is released into the synapse it is broken down by the enzyme acetylcholinesterase (AChE). Chemical inhibition of AChE increases the amount of ACh which is able to reach the receptor sites and thus improves reaction between ACh and receptors.

Edrophonium (Tensilon®) is a short-acting AChE inhibitor (anticholinesterase) that improves muscle weakness in most patients with MG by inhibiting the breakdown of cholinesterase. About 75% of myasthenics respond positively to Tensilon®, an injectable, quick-acting form of anticholinesterase, thus establishing a tentative diagnosis.

The test procedure is as follows: The physician determines which muscle group or groups are most severely affected, then the patient is instructed (or helped) to exercise that muscle group until weakness occurs. When weakness appears the Tensilon® is injected, usually into the vein at the inner elbow. The first injection is usually one or two mg. of a 10 mg. vial. If the patient does not react or does not experience an improvement in strength the remaining eight or nine mg. is injected. The strength of the muscle is then evaluated and compared to its pre-injection level.

Tensilon® begins to take effect in 30 - 60 seconds, reaches its peak of effectiveness in two to three minutes and wears off in five minutes. The patient is sometimes given an EMG, then given Tensilon® and the reaction recorded so that an objective, permanent record of the reaction is produced.

During a Tensilon® test the patient may feel some *side effects* like increased flow of saliva and tears, mild sweating, skin flushing, urinary urgency, abdominal cramping and twitching of the small muscles around the mouth.

It is quite possible for an MG patient to have a negative or indefinite Tensilon® test. Some patients do not respond to Tensilon® (just as some patients do not respond to anticholinesterases as treatment) but at times the testing procedure itself may be questionable. Several MG patients of the author's acquaintance report Tensilon® tests in which the muscles tested were not the muscles affected by weakness. Two patients reported the physician tested the grip when it was the legs or facial muscles that were affected. One patient had the legs tested when the upper body strength was compromised. Several reported that Tensilon® was injected without first exercising the affected muscles, resulting in little difference between pre- and post- injection strength. None of these patients responded positively, yet all eventually were diagnosed as myasthenic. Testing procedures are time consuming, expensive and at times uncomfortable. It is to everyone's advantage if they are carried out efficiently and correctly.

Neostigmine (Prostigmine®) may be used instead of Tensilon®. Neostigmine takes 15 - 30 minutes to take effect, reaches its maximum effect in about 40 minutes and may last up to three hours, which allows for a longer period of observation and testing.

These tests are not infallible. About 75% of MG patients respond positively to an anticholinesterase test but many do not. These drugs can also improve weakness in neuromuscular diseases other than MG.

These factors may confuse the issue if the clinician is inexperienced. Sinus bradycardia (a very slow heart rate), fainting, respiratory failure, seizure, severe abdominal cramping, diarrhea and nausea are all potentially serious side effects of the Tensilon® test. These side effects happen only very occasionally. However, for these reasons some neurologists prefer other tests.

## NOTES:

# 4

# HOW IS MG TREATED?

The first effective treatment for MG was the anticholinesterase drug Physostigmine®. Its use has now been supplanted by other anticholinesterases; neostigmine bromide (Prostigmine®) and pyridostigmine bromide (Mestinon®). These are the most frequently used treatment for MG. Mestinon® is the most widely used because it is least likely to cause side effects. Patients who do not respond well to Mestinon® may find Prostigmine® more effective.

The two drugs act in a similar way. When acetylcholine (ACh) floods into the synaptic cleft it immediately comes into contact with acetylcholinesterase (AChE). Acetylcholinesterase begins to break ACh down as soon as the two come into contact. Anticholinesterase drugs destroy AChE, prolonging the effectiveness of ACh, thereby enhancing neuromuscular transmission. These drugs do not cure MG, and only rarely do they restore completely normal functioning, but they do enhance the strength and endurance of weakened muscles. In most patients anticholinesterases will increase strength only up to a certain level. Increasing the dosage will not increase muscle strength any further. This level is called the maximum response. The maximum response level for each patient must be determined by careful adjustment of dosage and timing.

Mestinon® is available in several forms, including a liquid form for children or those with swallowing problems. There's a time release caplet called Timespan® (Supraspan® in Canada), which is primarily prescribed for those patients who have difficulty breathing at night, or who experience debilitating morning weakness. Timespan® allows these patients to sleep through the night without having to awaken to take medication. Timespan® releases at an inconsistent rate, so it is not recommended for daytime use and it should not be substituted for regular Mestinon®. The time release versions of these medications should never be crushed, as crushing allows all the medication to be absorbed immediately which can cause an overdose. They should also be stored in the original container with the supplied dessicant (drying agent) to avoid "mushiness".

It should also be noted that Timespan® is formulated using a variety of fillers and binders, one of which is zein, a protein synthesized from corn. Patients who have an allergy to corn should keep this in mind when taking the drug, as allergic reactions can sometimes mimic cholinergic (overdose) symptoms. There is at least one well-documented case where a patient repeatedly suffered severe overdose symptoms after taking Supraspan®, when an equal amount of Mestinon® provoked no such reaction. The manufacturer of Mestinon®, Timespan® and Supraspan® provided a complete list of the ingredients in Supraspan®, including the zein to which the patient had previously reacted violently in allergy tests. With this information it was possible to attribute the so-called overdose to an allergic reaction.

## SIDE EFFECTS

Some common side effects of the anticholinesterases include abdominal cramping, nausea, diarrhea, gas and increased production of both tears and bronchial secretions. The small muscles around the mouth and eyes may twitch. Some patients experience muscle cramps, especially in the feet. Muscle cramps are more likely to occur in patients who also take prednisone, which lowers potassium levels. These cramps can often be relieved by running hot water over the feet.

Side effects may be reduced by taking anticholinesterases with food, though patients who experience swallowing problems may need to take their meds 30 - 45 minutes before a meal to improve swallowing. Caffeine may increase muscle twitching. Taking anticholinesterases with citrus juice may cause an increase in gut cramping. If side effects become a major problem there are medications which can be prescribed to alleviate them, although some physicians are reluctant to use them because they can mask overdose.

The side effect that must be most closely monitored is an *increase* in muscle weakness which occurs an hour to an hour and a half after the medication is taken. An overdose of anticholinesterase can cause the patient to go into *cholinergic crisis* [22]though this is rare.

---

22 Cholinergic crisis: State caused by overdose of anticholinesterase medication. Symptoms include muscle weakness, twitching, increased salivation, sweating and constricted pupils.

A common starting dose of Mestinon® is 30 mg. three or four times daily, which may then be adjusted as needed. When adjusting dosages, either up or down, it is best not to change the amount by more than ½ a tablet (30 mg.) at a time. The danger of significant side effects is minimal with smaller doses and there is usually nothing to be gained by taking a dose of more than three tablets (180 mg.) at a time.

For those who have swallowing problems, Mestinon® tablets can be crushed and mixed with a small amount of smooth, easily swallowed food such as yogurt or soft custard. Crushed tablets should not be swallowed dry, since the powder can enter the lungs and cause serious respiratory problems. It is also possible to take Mestinon® by placing the tablet under the tongue and allowing it to dissolve. Some patients feel they get quicker response this way. If tablets prove to be a problem contact the nearest compounding pharmacy. A compounding pharmacy's specialty is preparing medications in forms which meet an individual patient's needs, such as a gelled Mestinon® syrup, which is less likely to cause choking in patients who have trouble swallowing pills or liquids.

Mestinon®'s side effects are short term and subside when the medication is discontinued. There is still some question about long term side effects. There has been speculation that extended usage may result in limited muscle atrophy, but this has yet to be proven, since the same kind of atrophy has been noted in long term MG patients who have not received anticholinesterases. The anticholinesterases remain the most used treatment for MG.

## BEGINNING ANTICHOLINESTERASE THERAPY

The patient who is just beginning anticholinesterase therapy may find it helpful to keep notes, recording the time and dosage of medication and the response. Some questions that could be asked are: Did the effect of the medication last a full four hours? If not, at what point did strength decline? Side effects such as twitching of the fine muscles around the eyes or at the corners of the mouth should be noted as should gut cramping or diarrhea. Notes such as these can be helpful in determining what level of medication should be the baseline and how much, if any, extra should be taken during times of physical or emotional stress.

Generally, patients begin by taking the prescribed dose every three to four hours. Adjustments to the dosage and timing can be made as the response becomes clear.

Dosages and schedules must be individualized. Most patients, once they have become accustomed to the medication and know how to read its effect, can take it on an adapted demand schedule. Not surprisingly, surveys have shown that myasthenics are the least likely of any patient group to forget their medication!

It can be very useful for the patient to do simple strength tests at home. The results can be noted and used by the physician to help determine effective dosage levels and timings. By comparing strength levels when the medication level is at its peak effect, and again when the effect is at its lowest level, it's possible to determine how much effect the medication is having. There is a form in the Appendix which can be photocopied and used to keep track of strength levels.

## STRENGTH TESTING

To do medication effectiveness testing start by testing strength at the end of a medication period when medication level will be at its lowest, or test first thing in the morning, before taking any medication. Test those areas which are affected by MG (the ability to hold up the arms, rise from a chair, breathe deeply, etc.). Don't overdo it or force muscles to work beyond their comfort zone. The idea is simply to evaluate strength.

To test the vital capacity (the amount of air held by the lungs), take a deep breath, exhale forcefully, take a second deep breath and then count clearly out loud, at a steady rate, as long as possible. An adult with good to excellent vital capacity should be able to count until they reach from 60 to 100. Note the number reached on the form, then repeat the sequence immediately. Note this number and do it a third time.

If the ability to hold up the arms is compromised, hold the arms straight out in front, or out to the sides, for as long as comfortable. Watch the second hand on the clock or have someone else keep time. Note the result on the form.

If neck weakness is a problem lie flat on a bed and lift the head free of the supporting surface. Count and note on the form.

To test leg strength sit on the edge of a chair and extend one leg straight out. Note the time you can hold the extension and record it.

To determine hip girdle strength count the number of times you can rise from a chair. For knee strength do knee bends. Ten in either case denotes excellent strength.

For those areas of weakness that are hard to measure, such as drooping eyelids, swallowing, talking or chewing, estimate on a scale of one to ten how strong these functions are with one representing severe weakness and 10 representing excellent strength.

None of these figures so far mean a great deal. It is only by comparing them with *medicated* strength that they assume significance. Repeat the series of tests at the peak of effectiveness of your medication (probably about one hour after a dose). Do the series of tests as closely as possible to the way you did them before. Note the results.

For example: Patient A has problems with compromised breathing ability. She did the breath test first thing in the morning before taking her first dose of Mestinon®. She was able to count to 62 with the first breath. With her second breath she was only able to reach 47. With her third breath she was only able to reach 32. An hour later, when her medication had reached peak levels, she did the three breath counting test with results of 65, 64 and 65.

This observed difference is an indication of the effectiveness of the medication. While observations of this kind are not 100% objective they can be very valuable when determining appropriate levels and dosages of the anticholinesterases. They can also help patients who experience a consistent daily or monthly pattern of fluctuating weakness to determine when they require more medication. Since dosage may vary from day-to-day depending on activity level, stress, infection or phases of the menstrual cycle, keeping track of predictable factors may help plan a medication schedule which will meet these needs.

## TREATING OCULAR SYMPTOMS

The most difficult symptoms to control are often the ocular ones; drooping eyelids, double vision and eye muscles which do not track properly. Ocular symptoms can be disabling, as they can prevent the patient from driving, reading or doing any work that requires visual acuity. Ptosis, or droopy lids, can affect one or both lids. If it becomes impossible to lift one or both eyelids ptosis crutches can be helpful. A ptosis crutch is a device mounted on the eyeglasses to hold the upper eyelid open. The patient has to remember to blink, because when the lid is held up with an artificial device, there's no automatic blinking and the eye can dry out.

Double vision is another very difficult symptom for many MG patients to deal with. Patching (with an eye patch or – more recently - by wearing an opaque contact lens on one eye) has frequently been used to treat double vision. Although patching eliminates double vision, the patient loses all depth perception and a large percentage of the field of vision. This results in an impaired ability to orient themselves in space. This may lead to problems with eye/hand coordination, clumsiness, bumping into objects and/or people, climbing stairs or curbs, crossing the street, driving and other activities of daily living which require depth perception and peripheral vision.

## FRESNEL PRISMS

Another option for treating double vision are thin plastic Fresnel prisms which are applied to the inside of both lenses of the patient's eyeglasses. A group of Swedish physicians reported that they were able to totally correct the double vision of almost half of the patients in their study with Fresnel prisms. A further 38% reported improvement. Thirteen percent of their patients did not respond at all, mostly elderly patients or those with severe problems.

## THE THYMUS AND THYMECTOMY

The thymus is a pinkish-gray mass of tissue located behind the sternum (breastbone). It lies over the trachea (windpipe). It is made up of many small lobes ranging in size from that of the head of a pin to a pea. The entire gland is covered with a tough membrane. The thymus activates components of the immune system and may affect other bodily functions as well. The thymus reaches its maximum growth by puberty. Beginning at about the age of 20, cellular material in the thymus gland gradually decreases in extent and is replaced by fatty tissue. This process is called *involution.* By the age of 60 years, 90% or more of the gland consists of fat.

The thymus appears to play a central role in the specific immune response which is responsible for MG. The autoimmune response to the AChR begins in the thymus when T cells produced in the bone marrow are activated there. Thymic overactivity (hyperplasia) or thymoma[23] is found in a high percentage of patients with MG.

---

23 Thymoma: Tumor of the thymus which is sometimes malignant.

Hyperplastic thymus in MG patients contain an increased number of B-cells. Some of these B-cells secrete anti-acetylcholine receptor antibodies.

Thymomas can be benign or malignant. The estimated frequency of thymoma in MG varies from 15 - 30%. It is more common with increasing age, with an estimated frequency of three percent for age 20 years or younger, 12% for ages 21 to 45, and 35% for age 46 years and older.

Surgical removal of the thymus, or *thymectomy*, has been a part of MG therapy since the 1930s. Response to thymectomy cannot be predicted with 100% accuracy. The occasional patient feels better almost immediately but most patients feel no improvement for months to years. Younger people who haven't had MG long seem to respond best to thymectomy, but some older patients gain significant benefit. In patients over 55 the thymus may have shrunk and the patient may not benefit from thymectomy.

Thymectomy is almost always performed on patients with thymoma. An exception might be in an elderly patient with a small thymoma, as thymectomy in these patients doesn't always improve MG symptoms.  Thymectomy is generally performed on all MG patients ages 10 - 55 years. It's reported that 40 - 60% of patients who have thymectomy go into remission within seven to ten years. Side effects of thymectomy are the same as for any major surgery; the risks of anesthesia, bleeding, and pain during recovery.

## THREE APPROACHES TO THYMECTOMY

There are three surgical approaches to thymectomy. During a trans-sternal thymectomy an incision is made lengthwise on the chest and the sternum is cut apart. The second method is called the trans-cervical. The incision is made immediately above the sternum, which is left intact. The third method (maximum thymectomy) involves making a cross-shaped incision and cutting through the sternum.

## PROS AND CONS OF EACH TYPE OF THYMECTOMY

The trans-sternal technique allows the surgeon to see the thymus and surrounding area, ensuring a more complete removal. However, the longer incision and separation of the sternum causes more post-operative pain and a longer recovery period than the trans-cervical technique.

The trans-cervical involves only a three or four inch incision. The sternum is undisturbed, so there is less post-operative pain and a quicker recovery. There is, however, a higher risk of missing some thymus tissue, and if bleeding becomes a problem it is harder to control. Some physicians feel that patients who respond poorly to trans-cervical thymectomy may do so because thymus tissue has been left behind. It's not unusual for thymus cells to grow onto the surface of adjoining organs. If this is the case it may be impossible to see through a small incision. Maximum thymectomy involves the largest incision. The sternum is split. Recovery time is longer than either of the other techniques, but since it opens the entire chest to the surgeon's view it is the method of choice if thymoma is suspected or discovered during surgery.

## COMPARING THYMECTOMY RESULTS

The following studies evaluated each method. Study number one followed 47 patients who had trans-sternal thymectomies. Study number two followed 72 patients who had maximum thymectomies. Study number three was conducted jointly at several medical centers around the world. It followed 1,242 patients who had a thymectomy, comparing the rate of relief from MG symptoms to the technique used.

### 1. TRANS-STERNAL (DUKE UNIVERSITY, DURHAM N.C.)
92% benefited
41% had complete remissions
23% had minimal symptoms controlled by medication
  7% were same as before surgery
One death

### 2. MAXIMUM (COLUMBIA MEDICAL CENTER, NYC)
96% benefited
46% had complete remission
33% had minimal symptoms
  4% same as before surgery
No deaths

### 3. TRANS-CERVICAL (MT. SINAI, ET AL.)
 (Remissions only noted)
 60% complete remissions (no discernible symptoms)

It is impossible to compare the results of these studies with total objectivity. Variables, such as the severity of each patient's condition, the length of time the patient had MG prior to the surgery and the age of patients must all be taken into account, but it is clear that many patients benefited.

The benefit of thymectomy to patients without thymoma is still a subject of debate. Recent studies conducted in different countries around the world have reported the following results.

In a study conducted at Laikon General Hospital, University of Athens, Greece, 76 Patients with MG underwent trans-cervical thymectomy. Twenty patients had thymomas (26%).

Results: Six months following surgery there was complete remission in 19 patients (25%), improvement in 49 (65%), no change in seven (9%) and impairment in one (1%) of the patients.

Five years following surgery the researchers were unable to contact 25 patients but of the 51 patients available for late follow-up, 19 (37%) were in remission. In 26 patients (51%) the symptoms had improved. In three (6%) symptoms were unchanged, and three (6%) had died of invasive thymoma at two and a half, three, and five and a half years after surgery. Patients who had symptoms for less than five years at the time of surgery, those who were in an earlier stage of disease, and those who did not have thymoma, had a better response.

At Nagoya City University Medical School, Japan, 375 patients with MG underwent maximal thymectomy. Surgeons opened the chest enough to allow removal of thymus tissue from fatty tissues adjacent to the lungs and from other organs in the chest. Of these patients, 89 had thymoma and 286 did not.

Reported remission rates in patients with thymoma were 13.6% (three months), 17.5% (six months), 27.5% (one year), 32.4% (three years), 23.0% (five years), 30.0% (10 years), 31.8% (15 years), and 37.5% (20 years).

Remission rates of patients without thymoma were 15.2% (three months), 15.9% (six months), 22.4% (one year), 36.9% (three years), 45.8% (five years), 55.7% (10 years), 67.2% (15 years), and 50.0% (20 years).

Factors which predicted a more favorable outcome were: The absence of thymoma, younger age and short duration of illness. Treating patients with steroids before surgery did not improve the outcome. Other studies reinforce the conclusions that the earlier the thymectomy the more likely the chance of achieving a full remission.

## WHO GETS A THYMECTOMY?

Most patients under age 60 who have generalized myasthenia of fairly recent onset are offered a thymectomy. Generally it has been felt that thymectomy was less likely to produce a full remission in patients with long standing cases, in patients over 60 or in those with very mild or strictly ocular symptoms. However thymectomy is now being offered to a wider range of patients, including those with only ocular symptoms.

In the thymectomy study quoted from Duke University, 14 of the the patients were over age 50, six were in their 60s, one was in his 70s and one was 82! One of these patients (age 60) died, one remained stable but unchanged, but all the rest improved, eight being either in remission or asymptomatic. The report on the study done at Columbia Medical Center does not give a breakdown of age in relation to improvement but patients ranged in age from 11 to 71 years. The conclusion might be drawn that although older patients might not be expected to improve as much as younger ones, they still may receive significant benefit. However, the risks of surgery are greater in older patients, and this is a factor which should be considered.

Thymectomy was once denied to patients who had MG symptoms longer than five years. This excluded many since some patients wait years for a diagnosis. The previously cited Duke University study included patients who had MG symptoms from one month to 34 years before diagnosis. Nine patients had symptoms five or more years. Two of these patients, with MG of seven years and 20 years duration respectively, did not improve after thymectomy. The rest improved, including four who became symptom free. These four patients had MG from five to 20 years before thymectomy. It appears that while the best results can usually be expected from timely surgery, thymectomy may benefit some patients who have had myasthenia for many years. Thymectomy is not without its detractors, but it is now a primary form of therapy for MG and is expected to remain so for many years to come.

## STEROIDS

The use of steroids has been reported to be of value in MG for almost 30 years, although they have been widely prescribed for only about 20 years. Corticosteroids (steroids for short) are man-made drugs which mimic the action of cortisol, a hormone produced by the adrenal glands. Cortisone, Prednisone® and methyl-prednisolone are all corticosteroids. They reduce the activity of the immune system by affecting the function of specific white blood cells. Steroids are frequently used to treat MG. Prednisone® is the most often used.

There are several different ways to administer steroids to the MG patient. Some physicians begin with a small dose and increase gradually. Others begin with a large dose and decrease it gradually. On alternate-day regimes the patient takes steroids one day and skips the next. A variation on the alternate-day regime has the patient take a larger dose of steroids one day and a small dose the next. When patients take steroids for longer than a month the dosage must be reduced gradually because steroid therapy suppresses the body's own production of natural steroids. A gradual decrease allows the adrenal glands to resume normal functioning and reduces the risk of a relapse of MG symptoms.

Generally, steroids are not prescribed unless the patient has not responded satisfactorily to anticholinesterases. In the previously cited study done at Mt. Sinai Medical Center (NYC), several conclusions were drawn. Since these drugs carry a substantial risk of toxic effects, including increased muscular weakness, it was recommended that steroids be prescribed only for patients with serious disabilities or life-threatening symptoms. This view is not universal.

The late Dr. T. R. Johns, Dept. of Neurology, University of Virginia School of Medicine, reported that, based on observations of 200 MG patients, he had concluded that steroid therapy is acceptable for any patient who presents more than mild non-progressive ocular or extremity (arms and legs) weakness. All patients with disabling MG symptoms (barring other major medical conditions that might be worsened by the drug) were prescribed steroids.

In the patients described by Dr. Johns dosages were begun at 60 - 80 mg. daily. As soon as the patient showed sustained improvement an alternate-day regime was begun. Then the dosage was slowly dropped until the lowest dose that would maintain improvement was reached.

All patients in the University of Virginia study were hospitalized to begin steroid therapy. Hospital records show that 48% of the patients experienced worsening symptoms during the initial treatment period. Though most of these symptoms were of mild intensity, 17.8% had weakness severe enough to require assistance with breathing, or required tube feeding. Some patients developed steroid-induced weakness within the first 24 hours of treatment, while others did not react for over two weeks. On average, steroid-induced weakness occurred by the fifth day of treatment.

Patients differed widely in the length of time the steroid induced weakness lasted. Some were weak only one day before improvement began, while a few had weakness that lasted for 20 days. The average period of steroid-induced weakness was slightly over four days. (It should be emphasized that the dosage of steroids these patients were initially given was high. The risk of this kind of early worsening of symptoms is much less when the initial dosages are small and are gradually increased.)

Improvement was noted after an average of 13 days. Some patients responded within 12 hours while others took a full 60 days. Eighty-five percent improved within three weeks. *Maximum improvement was achieved over a range of from two weeks to six years.* Most patients improved rapidly early in the treatment, and then continued to improve slowly, until maximum improvement was realized.

Some patients (14%) were able to eventually stop taking steroids and maintain their improvement. A slightly larger proportion (19%) required a small dose to maintain improvement. In these patients dosages ranged from five to 50 mg. on alternate days. Most required dosages on the lower side of that range. The rest of the patients were still being evaluated when the report was published, so their results were not included.

Several patient's symptoms grew worse. Almost half of these exacerbations were from reducing the steroid dosage too rapidly. About 25% were due to unknown causes. The rest followed pregnancy, major infection, surgery or carelessness about taking the medication. No patients developed sudden or severe weakness, all experienced a gradual deterioration of strength.

## SIDE EFFECTS OF STEROIDS

Sixty-six percent of the patients in this study developed some side effects. The common ones, "moon face" (cushingoid appearance), and weight gain were experienced by 33% and 18% of the patients respectively. These side effects were a problem primarily during the early (high dose) phase of treatment and resolved themselves when alternate-day, lower dosage therapy began. Twenty-six percent of the patients developed cataracts[24], 12% developed diabetes or high blood pressure. Osteoporosis (thinning of the bones) developed in nine

---

24 Cataracts: A condition in which the lens of the eye becomes cloudy or
    opaque.

percent, but only in those patients whose severity of symptoms led to long term (60 - 90 days) high-dosage therapy. There were some cases of increased susceptibility to infection (5%). Two percent of patients developed psychological disturbances. Two percent developed gastric ulcers and there was one case of glaucoma[25].

Steroid therapy carries an element of risk. Both patient and physician must carefully weigh expected benefits against the possibility of side effects in *that* patient. Factors such as family history, body type and pre-existing medical conditions must all be kept in mind when prescribing steroids.

One risk of long-term steroid treatment is thinning of the bone (osteoporosis). It is now routine in some clinics to prescribe medications like Fosamax® or Didrocal® (which are used to prevent and treat osteoporosis) if a patient is expected to take steroids longer than three months, which it almost always the case in MG therapy.

Because steroids suppress the immune system they make patients who take them more vulnerable to infection. They also can cover up the symptoms of infection. With long-term use of steroids the adrenal glands stop making corticosteroid hormones. For this reason steroid treatment must be stopped very gradually in patients who have taken it for more than a few weeks. This gives the adrenal glands time to "wake up" and begin producing their own hormone. If the drug is stopped too quickly, the patient may collapse from the lack of corticosteroid hormones. Patients taking steroids for longer than one month should carry a warning card for two years. In the case of an accident or illness they may need extra steroid to avoid shock.

Steroids also cause the excretion of potassium. Low potassium levels can cause muscle cramping, so patients should include potassium rich foods in the diet. Some reports have recommended that patients on steroids should be given low dose potassium therapy.

## MESTINON® AND STEROIDS TOGETHER?

In the past there were suggestions that anticholinesterases (Mestinon®, etc.) should be discontinued when a patient begins steroid therapy. Drs. R. G. Miller and H. S. Milner-Brown did a study at the University of California, San Francisco and Children's Hospital of San Francisco. This study involved 24 patients with varying degrees of myasthenic weakness. Measurements of strength were

---

25 Glaucoma: Increased pressure in the eyeball, which over time can lead to blindness.

taken at hourly intervals for two to six hours after the administration of Mestinon® alone, Mestinon® and Prednisone® combined and Prednisone® alone.

Patients administered Mestinon® alone improved by about 29% in muscle strength. Patients given the combination of Mestinon® and Prednisone® improved 60%. Patients given only Prednisone® did not experience an immediate improvement in strength. Based on this study it would appear that the drugs combined tend to be more, rather than less, effective.

It has also become the practice in most areas for steroid treatment to be initiated outside the hospital. Some neurologists feel that reports of worsened symptoms at the beginning of steroid treatment reflect the now largely-discarded practice of discontinuing a patient's anticholinesterase medication when steroid therapy was begun.

This is a somewhat difficult position to evaluate as many steroid studies reach back to a time period when this practice was common. This author could find only one study in which it was stated that all patients in the study were on anticholinesterases. This study compared the effectiveness of combined steroid and azathioprine (Imuran®) therapy to that of azathioprine alone. There were 89 patients in this study, 25 of which had respiratory compromise. Of these 89 patients, 32 were begun on azathioprine alone. Six of these 32 (18.76%) had respiratory compromise prior to the treatment. Of the 32 patients, 6.2% experienced a respiratory crisis which required the use of a respirator after initiation of therapy. Fifty-seven patients were treated with a combination of azathioprine and steroids. Of these, 19 (33.3%) had respiratory compromise prior to treatment. In this group, 29.8% had respiratory crisis which required a respirator after initiation of therapy.

In this study, almost all patients who had respiratory compromise experienced crisis when begun on the combination of azathioprine and steroids. Only five of the 89 patients were started on both drugs at once. The majority were begun on azathioprine only after they had not responded to steroids, or vice versa. When the rate of respiratory crisis in the patients receiving only azathioprine (6.2%) is compared with the rate of those who received steroids (29.9%) it becomes fairly obvious that the initiation of steroid therapy represents a substantial risk of crisis, especially in those with prior respiratory involvement.

We invited comment on this issue from eminent neurologist and author Dr. Donald B. Sanders, Professor of Medicine, Division of Neurology, Duke University Medical Center, Durham, North

Carolina. Dr. Sanders is the Director of the MG Clinic at Duke. He states:

> "If the patient is at significant risk for developing dysfunction of vital muscles (respiration or swallowing) he or she should be hospitalized for institution of high dose Prednisone® therapy. Patients with significant oropharyngeal[26] weakness are at greatest risk and those with predominantly ocular and mild generalized weakness probably at least risk. In addition to the severity of disease, however, must be considered the other factors that determine the safety of any therapeutic approach including how far away the patient lives and what medical facilities are available locally. Another factor is patient compliance. In an ideal situation, where the patient has demonstrated their ability to understand their disease and their willingness to call if any problems arise, it is reasonable to begin therapy outside the hospital. If there is any question about, this, however, the sagest approach is to have the patients hospitalized at least during the most crucial phase of Prednisone® therapy."

In view of such evidence, it seems prudent to admit patients in whom a worsening of symptoms could precipitate crisis, and to thoroughly instruct every patient beginning steroids to anticipate possible temporary worsening of symptoms. However this is much less of an issue in patients with milder symptoms and when beginning low-dose Prednisone®.

## THE CYTOTOXICS

The cytotoxic (immunosuppressant) drugs are now in widespread use in the treatment of MG. The most often used immunosuppressants are Imuran® (azathioprine), Cytoxan® (cyclophosphomide) and Cyclosporin A®. CellCept® (mycophenolate mofetil) is a newer immunosuppressant now prescribed to MG patients.

Azathioprine was originally used for long-term treatment of people with kidney transplants. The drug suppresses the immune system, thus preventing the body from rejecting the transplanted organ. Azathioprine is now also used to treat immune system disorders such as lupus and MG.

---

26 Oropharyngeal: Relating to the mouth and soft palate.

The immunosuppressants are not a first line treatment, though this is changing as many have fewer side effects than steroids. The immunosuppressants can cause a variety of side effects, depending on the drug. Some of these side effects are bone marrow depression, hair loss or increased hair growth, nausea and vomiting, fever, liver damage, bladder hemorrhages and sterility. There is also speculation that long term suppression of the immune system may increase the risk of malignancy, though this is yet to be proven. On the positive side there are researchers who feel that in the treatment of MG, where immunosuppressant drugs are given in lower doses than those given to transplant patients, they pose no more danger of toxic side effects than do steroids.

A German study involving 99 patients treated with azathioprine (for up to 10 years) reported that fewer than 10% had side effects requiring discontinuation of the drug. Other studies involving more than 800 patients came to the same conclusion. These researchers concluded that the adverse side effects seen in transplant patients do not apply to lower dose situations such as MG therapy.

## CYCLOSPORINE - A

Cyclosporine A® (CY-A) became available to MG patients in the early 1990s. It was used originally in organ transplant therapy but soon was found to be useful in treating autoimmune diseases.

The side effects of CY-A can include a rise in blood pressure, increased body hair growth, gut cramping and kidney damage. A more serious problem with long-term immune suppression is a rise in the malignancy rate. Studies show that MG patients treated with CY-A have an approximately 10% higher rate of malignancy.

Cyclosporine A® is a highly effective MG treatment. Patients not only improve while taking it, but are often able to discontinue their steroids. In one report of 57 patients who took CY-A for an average of three and a half years, 55 experienced clinical improvement and 38 were able to discontinue or decrease their dosage of steroids. Five percent of the patients who began the study stopped taking CY-A, either due to its cost or to side effects.

Cyclosporine A® should not be taken with grapefruit juice. Grapefruit juice inhibits an enzyme which metabolizes CY-A and can lead to an accidental overdose.

### CELLCEPT® - MYCOPHENOLATE MOFETIL

CellCept® is a newer immunosuppressant which appears to cause fewer side effects than other drugs in this class. It inhibits the production of B cells, including the antibodies involved in the autoimmune reaction in MG. CellCept® has become accepted as a therapy for MG, especially in cases where patients are resistant to other forms of therapy.

CellCept's® use in MG is first described in an article in the journal *Neurology* in 1998, when it was used to treat a man with severe MG who had responded to no other treatment. In the years since, a number of studies have been done evaluating CellCept's® effectiveness in treating severely affected MG patients who have proven difficult to treat.

### SUMMARY OF CELLCEPT STUDIES. (TABLE 4.1)

| Table 4.1 Study | #patients | #improved | side fx | quit drug |
|---|---|---|---|---|
| One: | 85 | 62 (73%) | 27.00% | 16.00% |
| Two: | 3 | 3 (100%) | 33.00% | 0.00% |
| Three | 12 | 8 (75%) | 0.00% | 0.00% |

Some patients responded to CellCept® in two weeks, while some took as long as eight months. Average response time was about three months. Dosages ranged from 1,000 to 2,000 mg. daily, which probably accounts for the differences in reports of side effects.

Side effects associated with the administration of CellCept® include diarrhea, low white blood-cell count, susceptibility to bacterial infection and nausea, but patients taking CellCept® may have a lower incidence of side effects than patients taking other immunosuppressants. Immunosuppressants are often used in conjunction with steroids, which results in improved effectiveness at lower dosages of each.

### PLASMAPHERESIS/PLASMA EXCHANGE

Plasmapheresis, now often called plasma exchange, is a frequently used treatment in MG. There is no controversy about its effectiveness, for there is no doubt that it is effective for the majority of MG patients, but there remains a wide variation in the criteria for its use.

In plasma exchange blood is drawn from the patient and passed through a centrifuge which mechanically separates the blood into several components. The plasma portion, containing the anti-AChR antibodies, is then subtracted and replaced with plasma or sterilized albumin separated from donor blood. From one to four liters of blood are treated in a typical exchange. Anticoagulants must be added to the blood as it is treated to prevent clots from forming. From four to eight treatments are usually required.

Plasma exchange is also used to treat myasthenic crisis, and to act as an interim supportive measure while waiting for steroids or immunosuppressants to take effect. The occasional patient who has severe MG responds to no other treatment. In these cases plasma exchange may be scheduled regularly to prevent life-threatening deterioration.

The patient usually feels well for three to six weeks following the procedure, then deteriorates to the previous level of disability. Patients with mild or moderate involvement are rarely considered candidates for plasma exchange, unless they are in crisis or facing surgery. The cost of plasma exchange is high and potential side effects (low blood pressure, reduced calcium levels, bleeding, infection, embolism and chest pain) occur infrequently but still must be considered. Plasma exchange has limitations but has proven to be a life saving adjunct to myasthenic care.

### INTRAVENOUS IMMUNOGLOBULIN (IVIG)

Human immunoglobulin (IgG ) is a product derived from human blood. IgG is one of five kinds of antibodies found in the body. IgG is a long-lived antibody that maintains control over infections after the other antibodies have fought the initial battles with invading bacteria or viruses. IgG antibody can be separated from whole blood, treated to remove any traces of bacteria or viruses, and then concentrated into a highly active form. Plasma from hundreds to thousands of donors is pooled to produce IVIG, which is administered intravenously in the same way IV fluids are given. For this reason the treatment is referred to as IVIG (IntraVenous ImmunoGlobulin). Patients are usually given two infusions daily over a two to five day period.

IVIG is used primarily as a treatment for MG patients in crisis, when it provides quick, but temporary, relief of symptoms for more than 75%. The patient usually feels well for three to six weeks following IVIG, then deteriorates to the previous level of weakness. IVIG is also occasionally used for long term management in seriously affected patients who cannot continue taking other medications due to intolerable side effects, but is rarely used in this way due to its cost.

There are few studies documenting IVIG as long-term therapy but one study described the use of IVIG in six such patients. All six patients received standard infusion of IVIG for five days (400 mg./kg./day). All the patients experienced improvement within a few days to a week. Their double vision went away and their strength improved. After the five day course of therapy, they were given 400 mg./kg./day once every three to four months. They were able to maintain their improvement while their prednisone and anticholinergic drugs were gradually withdrawn, and continued to receive IVIG maintenance dose at 400 mg./kg. once every three to four months. The patients in this study maintained their improvement for a minimum of 24 months only receiving IVIG as described above.

Complications sometimes arise when blood clots form in the vein used for the intravenous line. This is the most common serious side effect of IVIG therapy. Allergic reaction is another potentially serious side effect. In one study of 341 treatments, three serious side effects occurred, a clot in the jugular vein, an allergic reaction and a feeling of pressure behind the sternum. Treatment was discontinued in these three patients.

Side effects associated with administration of IVIG include mild headache, low-grade fever, chills, anemia, low back pain, nausea, a temporary drop in blood pressure and sweating. These side effects were mild and transient and most patients reported only one of them. Headache was the most commonly reported side effect. Side effects vary somewhat between brands of IVIG product, and some patients may tolerate one brand better than another. If side effects are a problem it may be worth discussing a change of brand with the physician. Infusion rates vary between brands, with recommended infusion rates for a 150 lb. (70 kg.) patient varying from about five to 12 hours.

IVIG may never become a first-line treatment, but it does give physicians an alternative for patients who respond to little else, or who have intolerable side effects to drugs which suppress the immune system.

### 3, 4 – DIAMINOPYRIDINE

The symptoms of Lambert-Eaton Myasthenic Syndrome (LEMS) and several of the congenital myasthenic syndromes (CMS) respond well to the potassium channel blocker 3, 4 - Diaminopyridine (DAP). DAP prolongs the duration of the action potential. This increases calcium entry into the nerve terminal, allowing more quanta of acetylcholine to be released from the vesicles.

Since the symptoms of LEMS and a number of CMS result from an inadequate amount of ACh being released from the nerve terminals, DAP is often very helpful in these patients. When DAP is combined with anticholinesterases about 80% of LEMS patients, and CMS patients of specific types, can improve substantially. Studies have shown that DAP is effective in treating both the motor and autonomic deficits of LEMS, increasing muscle force by up to 81%. Patients with some forms of CMS respond with a significant improvement in strength levels when treated with DAP.

DAP is taken orally, three to four times daily. The effect of the drug begins within about 20 minutes after a dose is taken. Side effects seem to be manageable by adjusting dosages. Some patients experience tingling sensations in the face, hands and feet, and around the mouth. DAP seems to increase, to some degree, the gut cramping caused by Mestinon®. The drug may also lower seizure thresholds in patients susceptible to seizure. In most patients, Mestinon® enhances and prolongs the effect of DAP, making it possible to take a smaller dose.

DAP has been designated an *orphan* drug in the US and is not commercially available in the U.S. That is, no major pharmaceutical company markets DAP. However the drug is available to appropriate patients by working with their physician. In many states DAP is available through compounding pharmacies. Compounding pharmacies provide special formulations of medications, like gelled Mestinon®, and drugs which have been approved by the FDA for use in rare conditions where therapeutic options are limited. DAP is available in some provinces, since it is used in Canada to treat MS.

### MONARSEN - A NEW THERAPY IN THE WINGS?

In 2003 Ester Neuroscience announced that they were working on the development of an entirely new type of therapy for MG. In the first quarter of 2004 the company received approval from the FDA to begin clinical trials for their product, called *Monarsen®*.

Monarsen® is in a new class of gene therapy drugs called antisense therapeutics. It is hoped that antisense therapies will revolutionize medicine in the next 20 years, but only time will tell whether they live up to their promise.

DNA is the genetic information for humans and almost every other living thing. The information contained in DNA is stored as a code which is made up of four chemical bases; adenine (A), guanine (G), cytosine (C), and thymine (T). These bases are arranged in sequences that specify how an organism grows and functions. DNA bases pair up with each other, A with T and C with G, to form units called base pairs. Each base pair is attached to a sugar molecule and a phosphate molecule. A unit consisting of a base pair, a sugar molecule and a phosphate molecule are called a nucleotide.

Monarsen® is a 20 base antisense nucleotide, which is stable enough to be taken orally as a liquid. It carries a genetic sequence which matches that of the gene which produces acetylcholinesterase (AChE). Monarsen® binds to a single portion of the gene which produces AChE and reduces the production of AChE. The amount required is very small, only 500 micrograms per kilogram (2.2 lbs) of body weight. Monarsen® has no cholinergic side effects, and no serious side effects have been identified in the small number of patients who have trialed it.

The therapeutic implications of this new drug are interesting. It might in time prove to be an alternative to Mestinon®, but many further trials will be required before it's possible to tell if Monarsen's® effectiveness in early trials can be safely duplicated in a wider population of MG patients.

## HOW THINGS HAVE CHANGED!

In less than 70 years the treatment of MG has been radically altered. Prior to 1934 there was nothing that could be done for the person who developed MG. Today we are armed with a variety of treatments. It is only in the last 20 years that it can be truly said that most MG patients will live a normal life span. While many MG patients will experience some degree of disability, gone are the days when the diagnosis of MG meant a shortened life or a life of immobility. Today many MG patients lead fairly normal, and sometimes extraordinary lives, all because of advances in treatment undreamed of only a few decades ago.

## NOTES:

# 5

# THE AUTOIMMUNE FORMS OF MYASTHENIA

We now know that what was once simply called myasthenia gravis (MG) is actually a whole group of related diseases which affect the neuromuscular junction (NMJ). We now understand enough about neuromuscular structure and function to classify the different myasthenias by antibody type, gene mutation or change in function.

In the past ten years knowledge about myasthenia has expanded tremendously. There has been speculation for years that other antibodies were at work in seronegative patients with acquired or autoimmune MG. Now, the identification of the MUscle Specific Kinase (MuSK) antibody has proven that a second antibody is responsible for a significant number of cases of MG, and the search continues to find other MG antibodies.

A few years ago there was limited understanding of the congenital (inherited) myasthenic syndromes, but in the last few years knowledge of the inherited myasthenias has virtually exploded. The inherited myasthenias will be discussed in Chapter Six.

## ACQUIRED OR AUTOIMMUNE MG

The most common type of MG is the acquired (autoimmune) form. This form is also referred to as *idiopathic* MG. *Idiopathic* means "cause unknown". No one knows why the immune system attacks the NMJ in autoimmune MG. The most commonly accepted theory is that the process begins in the thymus where the *myoid cells* are located. Myoid cells express[27] acetylcholine receptors (AChR). Myoid cells are surrounded by macrophages and helper T cells. If something goes wrong with a myoid cell it could lead to an autoimmune response.

---

27 Express: To manifest or produce.

There is also a hypothesis that MG could be triggered by a process known as *molecular mimicry*. In molecular mimicry, an immune response to an invading agent that resembles the structure of an AChR triggers the autoimmune response. The body recognizes its own tissues by means of small structures called *epitopes* which protrude from the surface of each cell. Every living organism has a unique epitope whose shape is recognized by that organism's immune system. This is the way the body distinguishes self from non-self. If the epitope of a cell has the correct shape, it is self. If it has the wrong shape, it's non-self. The molecular mimicry theory suggests that some segment of the invading agent's epitope might resemble the alpha subunit of the neuromuscular junction, and that the immune system mistakes the alpha subunits for the invader and attacks them, long after the real invader has been dealt with.

This theory is supported by the discovery that patients suffering from an autoimmune condition have antibodies to microorganisms that share an amino acid sequence with tissue affected by their disease. For example; some researchers suspected that the bacteria *myco-bacterium tuberculosis*, which shares an amino acid sequence with one component of cartilage,[28] might trigger an immune system attack on the cartilage itself. They cloned the sequence and injected it into rats, who then developed the autoimmune inflammation of the cartilage we call arthritis.

MG patients have a higher level of antibodies against a component of a bacterium called *Y. entero-colicca* than do unaffected subjects. This suggests that infective organisms may play a part in triggering autoimmune disease. It is unlikely that a single trigger would initiate an immune system disorder but a combination of triggers (bacterial agent plus genetic predisposition plus stress) might.

There's compelling evidence that the autoimmune response in MG originates in the thymus since 75 - 80% of MG patients have abnormalities of the thymus gland. Of that number 85% have thymic hyperplasia (an enlargement of thymus cells) and 15% have a thymoma[29].

The immune system doesn't seem to need much of a push to go awry and attack its own tissue. There is scarcely an organ or function that is exempt from immune system attack. Examples of immune system disorders are; rheumatoid arthritis, lupus, hypothyroidism (Hashimoto's thyroiditis), hyperthyroidism (Grave's disease), diabetes

---

28 Cartilage: the elastic tissue which covers joint surfaces.
29 Thymoma: a tumor of the thymus gland.

and Crohn's disease. Some people seem to have a genetic predisposition[30] to develop immune system disorders.

Autoimmune MG is not inherited directly, but a person's genetic predisposition may make them more likely to develop it or another autoimmune disorder. Only three to five percent of those with autoimmune MG will have a close relative with MG, but those with MG are likely to have close relatives with other kinds of autoimmune disorders.

Treatment of autoimmune MG is directed at suppression of the immune response or reducing the number of antibodies circulating in the blood.

## THREE TYPES OF AUTOIMMUNE MG

There are three types of autoimmune MG; 1) Anti-AChR Antibody MG, 2) Seronegative MG and 3) MUscle Specific Kinase (MuSK) positive MG. The most common type is Anti-AChR Antibody MG. These patients have identifiable antibodies to subunit alpha of the acetylcholine receptor site (the AChR). Anti-AChR antibodies are found in approximately 85% of MG patients who have generalized weakness, and 50% of those with Ocular MG.

Recently a new antibody has been discovered, the MUscle Specific Kinase (MuSK) positive antibody. The MuSK positive MG (MMG) patient has antibodies to the MuSK receptors in the NMJ. MuSK positive MG is found in about seven percent of MG patients.

About 10% of MG patients with generalized weakness clearly have antibody mediated MG but do not have identifiable antibodies. These patients are labeled *seronegative*. We know that these patients have autoimmune MG for three reasons; 1) They respond to plasma exchange therapy; 2) Injections of their serum cause lab mice to develop MG symptoms and; 3) Babies born to seronegative mothers sometimes develop transient neonatal myasthenia[31].

Let's look at the similarities and differences between these three types of generalized MG in detail.

---

30 Genetic predisposition: An inherited tendency
31 Transient neonatal myasthenia: temporary symptoms of myasthenia gravis caused by antibodies in the mother's blood passing into the baby's blood.

### ANTI-AChR ANTIBODY MG

Anti-AChR antibody MG is caused by the production of antibodies directed against the alpha subunit of the acetylcholine receptors, although the other subunits can be attacked as well.

## Mechanism of AChR antibodies in MG

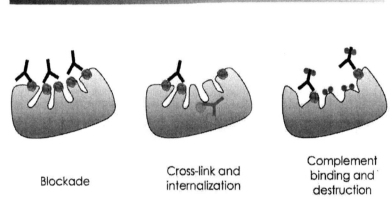

|          |                |                      |
|----------|----------------|----------------------|
| Blockade | Cross-link and | Complement           |
|          | internalization | binding and         |
|          |                | destruction          |

**Drawing courtesy M. Nicolle MD.**

Anti-AChR antibodies attack the AChR in three ways; they block acetylcholine binding sites, they bind AChRs and damage them, causing them to be absorbed into the muscle, and they bind complement and produce damage at the muscle endplate. This attack greatly reduces the number of available receptors sites. The antibody attack also causes structural changes in the NMJ, such as reduced folding of the muscle membrane and a wider gap between the nerve and the muscle.

In anti-AChR antibody MG the most typically affected muscles are the eyes, the muscles used for speech, swallowing and chewing, the face, arms, legs, neck, shoulders, hips and trunk. Occasionally, patients experience difficulty breathing due to weakness of the chest and diaphragm muscles. It is not unusual for symptoms to fluctuate from day-to-day or even during the course of a single day. Symptoms may be mild at first, and slowly increase in severity, or they may emerge with life-threatening rapidity within the space of days or weeks. This has led to a need for classifying symptoms in an organized way.

## MGFA CLINICAL CLASSIFICATION:

In 1997 the Medical Scientific Advisory Board of the Myasthenia Gravis Foundation of America (MGFA) formed a Task Force to develop a system of classification and outcome measures for myasthenia gravis (MG). In 2000, the Task Force published the MGFA Clinical Classification. This system divides MG into five classes.

**CLASS I:** Any ocular muscle weakness; may have weakness of eye closure; All other muscle strength is normal.

**CLASS II:** Mild weakness affecting other than ocular muscles. May also have ocular muscle weakness of any severity.

**IIA:** Predominantly affecting limb, axial muscles, or both. May also have lesser involvement of oropharyngeal muscles.

**IIB:** Predominantly affecting oropharyngeal, respiratory muscles or both. May also have lesser or equal involvement of limb, axial muscles, or both.

**CLASS III:** Moderate weakness affecting other than ocular muscles. May also have ocular muscle weakness of any severity.

**IIIA:** Predominantly affecting limb, axial muscles, or both. May also have lesser involvement of oropharyngeal muscles.

**IIIB:** Predominantly affecting oropharyngeal, respiratory muscles or both. May also have lesser or equal involvement of limb, axial muscles, or both.

**CLASS IV:** Severe weakness affecting other than ocular muscles. May also have ocular muscle weakness of any severity.

**IVA:** Predominantly affecting limb, axial muscles, or both. May also have lesser involvement of oropharyngeal muscles.

**IVB:** Predominantly affecting oropharyngeal, respiratory muscles or both. May also have lesser or equal involvement of limb, axial muscles, or both.

**CLASS V:** Defined by intubation, with or without mechanical ventilation, except when employed during routine postoperative management. The use of a feeding tube without intubation places the patient in class Ivb.

## TREATING AUTOIMMUNE MG

The goal of treatment in autoimmune MG is to reduce the level of anti-AChR antibodies and boost the level of ACh. This is done with a combination of therapies. Drugs remain a first line of defense. Anticholinesterase medications like Mestinon®, Prostigmine® and Mytelase® boost the level of ACh. Prednisone and other immune suppressants bring down the level of antibodies and stop or reduce the intensity of the attack.

A blood-filtering procedure known as plasma exchange (or plasmapheresis) removes harmful antibodies from the blood. The procedure known as intravenous immunoglobulin (IVIG) therapy infuses the patient with healthy antibodies which modulate the effects of the "bad" anti-AChR antibodies for several weeks. Finally, thymectomy (surgical removal of the thymus gland) is effective therapy for many patients. Each of these treatments is discussed in detail in chapter four on the treatment of MG.

## MuSK ANTIBODY POSITIVE MG

MUscle Specific Kinase (MuSK) is an enzyme essential to the formation of AChRs. MuSK and the protein *rapsyn* work together. They attract immature AChRs to the area beneath the nerve terminal, where under the influence of MuSK and rapsyn they cluster at the endplate, embed themselves in the NMJ and mature into working synapses. Anti-MuSK antibodies appear to impair neuromuscular transmission by blocking the clustering of AChRs into the NMJ. This results in an inadequate number of AChRs and reduces the communication between nerve and muscle, producing weakness.

Studies of MG patients in the *seronegative* group have revealed that 30 - 40% of them have MuSK antibodies. In MuSK positive MG (MMG) patients the immune system origin of the disease may be different than it is in anti-AChR antibody MG. The role of the thymus may be different too. So far, there have been no reports of any MMG patients with thymoma or thymic hyperplasia.

The number of reports on MMG are relatively limited, but it appears that this form of MG strikes women more frequently than men. Symptoms are reported as beginning at any time from childhood up to the seventh decade. Slightly over half of reported MMG patients developed the disease by the age of 40.

Some MMG patients have symptoms identical to the other forms of autoimmune MG but others have a different pattern of symptoms. If MMG patients have eye problems they develop later in the course of the disease. MuSK antibodies have never been found in a patient who has only ocular MG. Limb muscle weakness in MMG is less severe. More severe weakness is found in neck, shoulder and respiratory muscles. MMG patients tend to have a high frequency of respiratory crises. The course of MMG is often marked by exacerbations requiring hospitalization and assisted ventilation. Plasma exchange produces marked improvement in these cases.

## DIAGNOSING MMG

Tensilon® and Prostigmine® tests have been reported to be inconclusive or negative in a significant number of MMG patients. Single-fiber EMG (SFEMG) is the most sensitive exam for the diagnosis of MMG. One team used SFEMG to confirm 100% of the MMG cases they had identified by the presence of MuSK antibodies. However jitter may be abnormal *only* in muscles that are severely affected.

Electromyography (EMG) and Repetitive Nerve Stimulation (RNS) performed in limb muscles, are abnormal (positive) in 56.8% of cases. But RNS studies are frequently normal in limb muscles in MMG. However SFEMG, EMG and RNS studies will not identify the type of MG, they simply may reveal that there is an abnormality typical of MG. In MMG EMG findings may suggest myopathy, although myopathy may not show up on a muscle biopsy.

Diagnosing the MMG patient can be somewhat difficult, but a serological test[32] is now available to physicians. In the Americas call Athena Diagnostics at: 800 – 394 - 4493. Athena Diagnostics has a website at: http://www.athenadiagnostics.com/. Type MuSK in the search box.

European physicians who want a patient tested for MuSK antibodies should contact:
Prof Angela Vincent,
Neurosciences Group,
Weatherall Institute of Molecular Medicine,
John Radcliffe Hospital,
Oxford OX3 9DS England

---

32 Serological test: Looks for antibodies against MuSK in the patient's blood serum.

## MMG TREATMENT

Anticholinesterase medications produce a variable response in MMG. Like patients with anti-AChR antibodies, MMG patients may improve after plasma exchange, and many respond well to early, aggressive immune-suppressant therapy. In studies of MMG patients who've had a thymectomy, the thymus was normal or atrophied, and the surgery was of no benefit. Most knowledgeable neurologists now advise against thymectomy for MMG patients.

## SERONEGATIVE MG

Myasthenia gravis patients who have no detectable anti-AChR or MuSK antibodies are given the diagnosis of *Seronegative MG* (SNMG). Evidence for the role of antibodies in seronegative disease can be demonstrated by transferring MG symptoms to mice through an infusion of the patient's IgG. The target of the immune system attack in SNMG hasn't been identified, but it's only a matter of time, given the number of research teams who are working on the problem.

In SNMG the autoimmune attack increases AChR breakdown and reduces AChR function. Blood plasma and non-IgG immune fractions[33] from SNMG patients contains an immune factor, perhaps an IgM antibody, that inhibits AChR function but it is not clear how this factor works. Studies have shown that this as yet unidentified plasma factor in SNMG patients, distinct from MuSK IgG antibodies, binds to a muscle membrane receptor and activates a second messenger pathway leading to AChR breakdown and reduced AChR function.

## TREATMENT OF SERONEGATIVE MG

Seronegative MG is treated the same as autoimmune MG, with the exception of thymectomy. When the patient has no anti-AChR antibodies, thymectomy is usually not performed since experience has taught that thymectomy is generally of no benefit. Seronegative patients may require a treatment regime tailored just for them, because they may not respond to a typical course of treatment.

---

33 See Chapter 1 for explanation of immunoglobulins.

## OCULAR MG

Twenty to twenty-five percent of MG patients have a form of the disease known as *Ocular* Myasthenia. In ocular MG symptoms remain confined to the muscles which control the movements of the eye and eyelids. The pupil is not involved. There is blurred or double vision, drooping eyelids, weak eye closure, a "bouncing" movement to the eyes when the gaze is forced to the side, and an inability to move the eyes up, down, or to the right or left as needed.

Ocular muscle weakness is the first symptom most MG patients experience but within two to three years most patients with ocular symptoms go on to develop generalized myasthenia. This is probably because anti-AChR antibodies attack AChRs in neuromuscular junctions of skeletal muscle in all areas of the body, but even the slightest weakness in ocular muscles can cause problems with vision, and thus weakness is apparent first in the eye muscles. True ocular MG is usually not designated as such until the patient has had *only* ocular symptoms for a period of at least two years.

Estimates vary but from 50 – 85% of patients who begin with ocular symptoms eventually develop weakness in other areas of the body. Anti-AChR antibodies are found in 50 - 70% of patients with long-term, strictly ocular, symptoms. This is a significantly lower rate of anti-AChR antibodies than found in patients with generalized symptoms, but research suggests that this may be due to the fact that the antibodies responsible for ocular MG attack the AChR and bind to the epsilon subunit, rather than the alpha subunit.

The lower rate may also reflect the insensitivity of the anti-AChR antibody test. A newer, more sensitive, test recently detected anti-AChR antibodies in 17 of 110 ocular MG patients who had previously been found antibody negative.

Having symptoms localized to the eyes does not mean there's no chance of thymoma, though the risk is less if the patient has no anti-AChR antibodies. Every patient with ocular MG should have a CT scan of the chest to rule out any involvement of the thymus gland, as well as a thyroid workup to rule out Grave's disease.

## OCULAR MG OR EARLY GENERALIZED MG?

Though many patients with *generalized* MG experience weakness of ocular muscles as their first symptom, it may take one or more years after ocular symptoms appear for generalized weakness to develop. Under these circumstances how does the physician tell early-stage generalized MG from ocular MG? Since the ocular MG patient can have Anti-AChR antibodies, physicians usually assumed a "wait and see" approach. Patients were treated with anticholinesterases and an eye patch. If the double vision was disabling small doses of prednisone were prescribed.

In the mid-1990s some neurologists realized that many patients initially diagnosed with ocular MG developed generalized MG within one to four years. They theorized that many so-called ocular patients must actually be in the early stages of generalized MG. They wondered if early aggressive treatment could prevent them from developing generalized MG later on. With that in mind, studies were done comparing patients with ocular MG who were treated aggressively with those who were given more conventional treatment

**RESULTS OF AGGRESSIVE IMMUNOSUPPRESSANT THERAPY ON EARLY OCULAR MG SYMPTOMS (TABLE 5.1) Abbreviations:** GMS=Generalized Myasthenic Symptoms; Dip=Diplopia (double vision)

| Study | Untreated | Treated | Treatment | Response | Time |
|---|---|---|---|---|---|
| 1 | GMS developed in 13 of 36 | GMS in 4 of 58 treated | 40 – 60 mg/d prednisone then tapered dose | Incidence of GMS reduced from 36% to 7% | Two years |
| 2 | No untreated patients | Dip reduced from 29 of 32 to 8 of 32. GMS in only 3 of 32 | 40-80 mg/d prednisone tapered off over 4-6 weeks | Incidence of GMS reduced by 40% | Two years |
| 3 | GMS developed in 10 of 29 | GMS in 3 of 27 | 60-mg/d prednisone tapered off over 3 months | Incidence of GMS reduced from 34% to 11% | Two years |

## TREATMENT OF OCULAR MG

While ocular symptoms may not be life threatening they can be the forerunners of more serious symptoms. There is no reliable way to tell whether ocular symptoms will remain localized or develop into generalized MG. Unfortunately, ocular symptoms don't usually respond well to anticholinesterases. Prednisone® or azathioprine (Imuran®) appear to be the most effective treatments. Anti-AChR antibody positive ocular MG is now also being treated with thymectomy, although this approach is still controversial.

Follow-up studies of ocular MG patients revealed that remission rates increased gradually over time in patients who had thymectomy. One study followed 22 patients and quoted a remission rate of 11.8% at three years, 23.1% at five years and 33.3% at 10 years.

The most important factor influencing rate of remission appeared to be the duration of illness before thymectomy was performed. The longer the patient had been ill before surgery the longer it took for remission to occur. But only one patient of the 22 (4.5%) developed generalized MG later. Another study followed 14 patients with ocular MG who underwent thymectomy. Nine of these patients eventually went into remission, three improved significantly, and two improved somewhat. No patient became worse, and none died. The remission rates at one, three, five and ten years after surgery were 50.0%, 58.3%, 60.0% and 80.0%. Rates of improvement at one, three, five, and ten years after the surgery were 64.3%, 75.0%, 80.0% and 100%.

Patients who had shorter duration of illness before surgery obtained improvement and remission more quickly than patients who had been ill longer. Those who had been ill the longest (over seven years) were the ones who failed to obtain remission. In patients who had thymectomy those with ocular MG obtained remission more quickly than patients with generalized MG.

## LAMBERT-EATON MYASTHENIC SYNDROME

Lambert-Eaton Myasthenic Syndrome (LEMS) is a rare disorder, found only in about one of 100,000 persons. It's slightly more common in men than in women. It's uncommon for a patient to develop LEMS under the age of 30. When a child develops symptoms of LEMS the possibility of Congenital Myasthenic Syndrome, whose symptoms resemble those of LEMS, should be considered[34].

---

34 See chapter six; The Congenital Myasthenic Syndromes.

LEMS is similar to MG in that they both are the result of autoimmune attacks on the neuromuscular junction. The difference between them is the site of the attack. In MG the acetylcholine receptors are attacked. In LEMS the immune system attacks primarily the P/Q calcium ion channels on the nerve terminal. The P/Q calcium channels control the release of acetylcholine from the nerve terminal. In LEMS the immune-system attack on these ion channels reduces the amount of ACh released.

Patients with LEMS experience weakness of voluntary muscles. Their strength may improve when they exercise for a brief time, but weakness returns if they continue exercising. This aspect of the disorder is used as an aid in diagnosis. During vigorous exercise in normal skeletal muscle, the compound muscle amplitude potential (CMAP) rises by 20%. If the muscle is rested for 30 minutes immediately afterwards the CMAP falls back to normal. In a person with LEMS the CMAP may rise by 100% immediately following exercise, then fall to below normal strength during rest.

In addition to muscle weakness, LEMS patients may also have problems like dry eyes and mouth. They produce too little sweat, have difficulties with urination and experience severe constipation. Men with LEMS also may experience impotence and erectile dysfunction. Patients may have a pins and needles sensation in the hands and feet and almost always have reduced or absent deep tendon reflexes. The pupils of their eyes may react slowly to light. They frequently have blood pressure abnormalities.

These problems occur because the immune system attack on the P/Q calcium channels affects the release of ACh, not only at the axon terminal but at the junction of other nerves and tissues as well, such as the junction of the autonomic nerves and the tear duct, the salivary gland, the mucus membranes etc.

Most LEMS patients with cancer are smokers or have a long history of smoking. The P/Q form of LEMS occurs in 0.4% to 3% of lung cancer patients. LEMS symptoms usually precede the diagnosis of cancer by six months to five years. About 50% of P/Q LEMS patients (70% of the men and 39% of the women) eventually develop cancer of the lung. For some reason this ratio is changing. Fewer LEMS patients than before are developing lung cancer and more cases are of the autoimmune form. This may be because smoking is less popular, and there is less lung cancer and the associated P/Q LEMS.

It's believed that voltage-gated calcium channels (or a similar protein) on the surface of lung cancer cells in lung tumors may initiate an autoimmune cascade which attack the P/Q calcium channels on nerve terminals and results in LEMS. The calcium-channel subtype (in the tumor) which is responsible for the attack is not yet known.

LEMS patients show characteristic changes on EMG and nerve conduction studies (NCS), a lower than normal CMAP amplitude and decrement on repetitive nerve stimulation (RNS). More than 90% of LEMS patients also have anti-voltage gated calcium channel antibodies. Deep tendon reflexes are also greatly reduced or absent.

The muscle weakness in LEMS and MG is very similar, but the development and pattern of distribution tend to be different. The general rule is that, in MG, symptoms begin in the eyes and descend, while in LEMS, symptoms begin in the legs and ascend. This pattern can help physicians tell the difference between MG and LEMS. One group of researchers compared the patterns of weakness in 101 patients with MG and 38 with LEMS. A diagnosis of LEMS can be almost completely excluded in patients whose first symptom is ocular weakness. It was also noted that weakness confined only to the arms is seen only in MG.

## DIFFERING PATTERNS OF WEAKNESS IN MG & LEMS. (TABLE 5.2)

| Table 5.2 | | | |
|---|---|---|---|
| Initial Symptoms MG | Initial Symptoms LEMS | Maximum Severity MG | Maximum Severity LEMS |
| extraocular[35] muscles 59% | ocular muscles 0% | purely ocular in 25% | purely ocular 0% |
| bulbar muscles 29% | bulbar muscles 5% | ocular + bulbar in 5% | only bulbar 0% |
| limb muscles 12% | limb muscles 95% | limbs only 2% arms only 12% | legs affected 100% |
| | | ocular +bulbar + limbs 68% | |

---

35 Extraocular: any of six small voluntary muscles that control the movement of the eyeball.

## THERAPIES FOR LEMS

When a LEMS patient has cancer, treatment of the cancer will sometimes help resolve the LEMS. This is difficult to assess since most LEMS patients who improve as their cancer is treated are also treated with Prednisone® and chemotherapy. Prednisone® is used alone or in combination with other therapies. Most LEMS patients benefit from Mestinon® and 3,4 – Diaminopyridine. (DAP). DAP inhibits potassium channels in the nerve. This prolongs nerve depolarization and allows more calcium to enter the nerve through the voltage-gated calcium channels. The nerve then releases more ACh. Cyclosporine A and azathioprine are used cautiously when a LEMS patient has cancer, since they can reduce the body's ability to fight off the cancer. Thymectomy is of no benefit in LEMS.

If weakness is disabling, plasma exchange or IVIG may provide quick, short-term relief. One trial reported significant improvement in limb strength when LEMS patients received infusions of IVIG compared to patients who received placebo infusions. This improvement in strength lasted for up to eight weeks.

## DRUG-INDUCED MG

MG occasionally develops in patients treated with the drug D-Penicillamine (D-Pen). D-Pen (not to be confused with penicillin) is prescribed for rheumatoid arthritis, Wilson's disease (a metabolic disorder that affects copper excretion) and for some types of kidney stones.

D-Penicillamine-induced MG (DMG) symptoms usually appear within a few months of starting treatment with D-Pen. Symptoms disappear within three to six months after the drug is discontinued. Patients with DMG may have anti-AChR antibodies, so DMG can be clinically indistinguishable from autoimmune MG. Symptoms may become life-threatening, requiring aggressive therapy, including plasma exchange and immune suppression. The only way to determine if D-Pen is actually inducing the myasthenia is to discontinue it and wait and see.

In one report, five of 71 rheumatoid arthritis patients who received D-Pen developed autoimmune MG within a two-year period. When considering use of D-Pen physicians must make patients aware that MG is a possible side effect. Both patient and physician must remain vigilant for even minor initial myasthenic symptoms, and immediately stop the use of D-Pen if MG symptoms occur.

# 6
# THE CONGENITAL MYASTHENIC SYNDROMES

The congenital myasthenic syndromes (CMS) are a group of rare inherited disorders which affect neuromuscular transmission. It's only been in the past twenty years that the CMS have been widely recognized and described by medical science. The CMS are so rare that in some forms only a single patient has been described in medical literature. This means that descriptions of these forms of CMS are still very basic, and knowledge about them is extremely limited.

The congenital myasthenias are caused by genetic errors which cause malfunctions in one or more areas of the neuromuscular junction. While it's possible for a CMS to arise as a result of a spontaneous mutation (i.e. a birth defect), mutations are often inherited. In other words, they are passed from parent to child. They can be passed in an *autosomal dominant* pattern, which means only one parent need carry the affected gene, or they may be passed in an *autosomal recessive* pattern, which means both parents must carry the gene. In most cases, parents are totally unaware of the risk for CMS until one of their children is diagnosed. In some cases one or more children in a family has died without a diagnosis before CMS is finally recognized.

## THE CELL

The human body has more than 200 different kinds of cells. They provide structure for the body, absorb nutrients from food, convert those nutrients to energy and regulate the temperature of the body. Cells also contain the body's hereditary material and can duplicate themselves.

Cells could be called living machines. A cell has many parts, each with a different function. Some of these parts perform specific tasks. The *plasma membrane* is the cell's outer skin. It holds the cell together. The membrane is pierced by ion channels (pores) which control the flow of ions of sodium, calcium and potassium in and out of the cell.

The nucleus of the cell contains the genetic information needed to reproduce an identical copy of the cell. Every living thing, from bacteria to blue whales, has its own unique genetic blueprint (referred to as a genome). The genome is encoded in deoxyribonucleic acid (DNA) organized into units called genes.

## GENES, INSTRUCTION MANUALS FOR LIFE

The gene is the basic unit of heredity. Working from genetic instructions, molecules assemble into proteins and then into organs and tissues. The Human Genome Project has estimated that humans have between 30,000 and 40,000 genes.

Humans have two copies of each gene, one inherited from each parent. While more than 99% of human genes are the same in everyone, a small number vary slightly from person to person. Many of these have to do with physical differences such as eye and skin color, the size and shape of body and facial features, etc. These differences contribute to each person's unique physical appearance.

## CHROMOSOMES

The DNA molecule is packed into thread-like structures called *chromosomes*. A normal human cell has 23 pairs of chromosomes for a total of 46. Twenty-two of these pairs, called *autosomes*, are the same in males and females. Pair 23 are the sex chromosomes. They are different in males and females. Females have two copies of the X chromosome, while males have one X and one Y.

## A LIVING CODE

For the body to function properly the proteins in our cells must work flawlessly. Occasionally, a genetic mutation will prevent one or more of these proteins from forming and/or working properly. When a genetic mutation[36] affects a protein that plays a vital role in body function a *genetic disorder* can result.

---

36   Mutation: A permanent change in a gene which alters the trait or
     function expressed by the gene.

The genetic information for almost every living thing is stored in DNA. DNA is a living database which uses four chemical bases: adenine (A), guanine (G), cytosine (C), and thymine (T) as its alphabet.

The order (or sequence) that these bases are arranged in specifies how the organism develops and how it will function. Human DNA contains about three billion of these chemical bases. More than 99% of these bases are identical in every person in the world.

DNA bases team up with each other, A with T and C with G, to form units called base pairs. Each base pair is attached to a sugar molecule and a phosphate molecule. This unit, consisting of the base pair, a sugar molecule and a phosphate molecule, is called a nucleotide.

Nucleotides are arranged in two long strands that form a spiral called a *double helix*. The double helix looks something like a spiral staircase, with the base pairs forming the rungs and the sugar and phosphate molecules forming the vertical 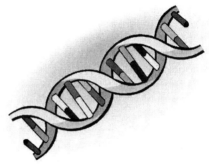 supports. It is an elegant and beautiful structure but the most important thing about DNA is that it can make copies of itself. This is critical because when a cell divides the new cell must contain an exact copy of the DNA which was present in the old cell. The strand divides down the middle and reproduces itself exactly in a new cell.

## How Cells Divide

Cells divide in two ways: by *mitosis* (my-toe-sis) or by *meiosis* (my-oh-sis). Mitosis is used to make new body cells. During mitosis a cell grows an exact copy of itself and then splits in half. Each new cell is exactly like the parent cell, with 46 chromosomes (two pairs of 23).

Meiosis is cell division that creates an egg or sperm cell. Sperm and egg cells each carry only 23 chromosomes - so meiosis, the process which creates sperm and egg cells, is a two-step process. The parent cell duplicates itself and then splits into two identical cells carrying 46 chromosomes. Those two cells then divide again, each producing two eggs or two sperm. This division reduces the number of chromosomes in each cell from 46 to 23.

When a sperm and egg cell unite at conception each carries 23 chromosomes, resulting in the 46 necessary for the new life. Meiosis creates genetic variation by shuffling DNA while the cells are dividing. Every person has two copies of every gene, one inherited from each parent. During meiosis one copy of each gene goes into the sperm or egg. This gene will then contribute to the new child's genetic makeup.

## GENETIC MUTATIONS

A *genetic mutation* is a permanent change in the DNA sequence that makes up a gene. Genetic mutations occur in two ways. They can be *inherited* from a parent or *acquired* during a person's lifetime. Inherited mutations affect almost every cell of a person's body since they are changes to the original cells that create the body. Acquired mutations are changes to the DNA of individual cells which happen during a person's lifetime. Acquired mutations can be caused by factors such as exposure to toxic chemicals or sunburn. They can also occur if the DNA makes a mistake as it copies itself during cell growth and division. These mutations do not get passed to the next generation unless they occur in the egg or sperm cell. If a mutation occurs in an egg or sperm cell there is a chance that it will get passed to the next generation.

## DOMINANT AND RECESSIVE INHERITANCE

Genetic traits are inherited in a number of patterns, but we will discuss only two of them, the *autosomal dominant pattern*, and the *autosomal recessive pattern*. All of the congenital myasthenic syndromes identified to date appear to be inherited in one of these two patterns, autosomal dominant, or autosomal recessive.

## AUTOSOMAL DOMINANT TRAITS

Only *one* copy of a mutated gene is needed for a person to inherit an autosomal dominant disorder. An affected person usually has one affected parent. Either males and females can inherit the mutation, and can pass the mutated gene equally to male and female offspring. Each child conceived by a set of parents (one of whom has the autosomal disorder) has statistically a 50% chance of inheriting the gene. In any one particular family these statistics may not be apparent, due to the small number of individuals. In some families fewer than 50% of children will inherit, in other families more than 50% will inherit.

Autosomal dominant CMS can also be caused by a sporadic (or new) mutation. Sporadic cases might be classified as genetic accidents. The number of cases caused by sporadic mutations is unknown. There is no behavior, diet or outside factors we are aware of which influences inheritance of autosomal dominant genetic disorders, other than the genes themselves, and chance.

## AUTOSOMAL RECESSIVE TRAITS

*Two* copies of the mutated gene must be inherited for a person to be affected by an autosomal recessive disorder. An affected person usually has two unaffected parents who each carry a single copy of the mutated gene. Persons who carry the mutated gene but are not themselves affected are referred to as carriers. Recessive disorders may be more difficult to identify and diagnose unless a family has two or more members who inherit the disorder.

## GENETIC ILLNESSES ARE NO CAUSE FOR SHAME

It's important for those who have a genetic disorder in the family to know that there is no reason to feel shame or guilt. There are no factors, such as diet, income level, race, religion or social class, which cause inherited diseases. There is absolutely *no evidence* that the congenital myasthenic syndromes can be caused (or prevented) by the actions of parents or grandparents. We have no idea why mutations occur or how to prevent them. Now that we know more about the human genome we've come to realize that everyone has at least one or two genetic mutations, but most of them have little or no impact on health.

## WHAT ARE THE SYMPTOMS OF CMS?

The congenital myasthenias cause muscle weakness and fatigability similar to those of MG. The symptoms of CMS usually begin within the first two years of life, although in a few forms patients can develop their first symptoms as late as the seventh decade of life.

### THE DIAGNOSIS OF CMS IS SUGGESTED BY THE FOLLOWING:

- Onset of symptoms in infancy or childhood.
- Weakness which increases as muscles tire.
- A decremental EMG response, on low frequency, of the compound muscle action potential (CMAP).
- No anti-AChR or MuSK antibodies.
- No response to immunosuppressant therapy.
- Family history of symptoms which resemble CMS.

The symptoms of CMS vary from mild to severe, depending on the form. It's also common for patients with the same form, even members of the same family, to be affected to differing degrees. In most forms of CMS weakness does not progress, and in some forms symptoms may diminish as the patient gets older. Only rarely do symptoms of CMS become worse with time.

In some forms of CMS symptoms begin before birth. In such cases the fetus is likely to be very quiet and move little in the uterus. Ultrasound exams may reveal that the fetus has abnormally flexed or extended limbs, and there is often too much fluid in the uterus.

An infant with CMS is likely to have a problem nursing. The infant may tire rapidly when feeding, choke frequently, have a weak cry, eyelid ptosis and generalized weakness. There may be times when an affected infant cannot breathe adequately without assistance. Infants with CMS may sit, crawl and walk later than unaffected infants of a similar age. They may develop aspiration pneumonia[37] from choking and inhaling food or their own secretions.

Children with CMS usually experience increasing weakness with sustained exertion. This is referred to medically as *fatigability*. They tire quickly when they are active and often have difficulty running, climbing stairs, jumping or doing any active repetitive movement. They often have trouble keeping up with other children. They may have fluctuating eyelid ptosis and external ophthalmoplegia[38]. They may develop postural scoliosis[39] when standing due to weak back muscles. In some cases muscle atrophy (wasting) may occur.

---

37 Aspiration pneumonia: Pneumonia caused by inhaling food, liquid, body secretions, etc.
38 External ophthalmoplegia: Limitation of eye movements; the eye is unable to look up, down or inwards.
39 Postural scoliosis: A curve in the spine which develops or worsens as trunk muscles tire while standing or sitting.

## TESTING FOR CMS

### LAB TESTS

In patients with CMS the blood level of creatine kinase (CK) may be normal or slightly elevated. Creatine kinase is an enzyme in muscle cells which aids energy production. When muscle cells are damaged the walls break open and the contents of the cell spill out, eventually making their way into the bloodstream. When this happens the CK level in the blood rises which can be an indication that muscle damage is occurring or has occurred recently. The CK level is measured with a simple blood test. Those scheduled to have blood drawn for a CK test should limit exercise to normal activities before the test.

### EMG TESTING

Patients will usually be tested for a decremental EMG response of the Compound Muscle Amplitude Potential (CMAP) at a low-frequency (2 - 3 Hz). If there is no decremental response from the lower level of stimulation the stimulation is usually turned up to 10 Hz, and the muscle is stimulated for a longer period of time. If the patient has CMS this stronger stimulation will usually lead to a significant decremental response. Single-fiber EMG is an alternate test to the CMAP and often the most accurate test available for CMS.

### MUSCLE BIOPSY

Conventional muscle biopsies usually show no major abnormalities, other than minor myopathy[40] and Type I fiber predominance. A few research centers do more detailed studies on endplates which allow a more precise diagnosis.

### GENETIC TESTING

The cause of many cases of CMS has been traced to mutations in the genes for the acetylcholine receptor (AChR) subunits. These mutations are located on chromosomes 2 and 17. Through genetic analysis of genes associated with CMS the underlying mutation may be identified in a high proportion of patients. Genetic testing is still an area of research and is not yet available on a commercial basis.

---

40 Myopathy: Muscle weakness or loss.

Several gene mutations have been identified with CMS. These include mutations in the genes encoding the five subunits of the acetylcholine receptor; two alpha subunits; and one each for beta, delta, and epsilon subunits; mutations in the gene encoding the collagen-like tail subunit of acetylcholinesterase; mutations in the gene encoding choline acetyltransferase; and mutations in the gene encoding rapsyn.

## THE DIFFERENT FORMS OF CMS

The congenital myasthenic syndromes are caused by a range of genetic errors that affect the structure and function of the NMJ. Grouped by the location of the defect, these abnormalities include:

### PRESYNAPTIC:

- Defects in the production, storage or release of acetylcholine.

### SYNAPTIC:

- A deficiency of acetylcholinesterase, the enzyme which breaks down acetylcholine in the synaptic cleft.

### POST-SYNAPTIC:

- Too few acetylcholine receptors.
- Slow channel syndromes in which the ion channel is slow to close.
- Fast channel syndromes in which the ion channel closes too quickly.
- Mutations which affect the function of the AChR sites. Some affect the ability of the AChR sites to bind to ACh. Others make ACh bind to the site too long. Finally, some mutations make the AChR site stay open, and some make it stay closed.
- Rapsyn mutations: Rapsyn works with MuSK to cluster AChRs at the NMJ. The mutations cause diminished clustering of AChR.
- A Sodium channel mutation: Results in a failure to trigger action potentials. The mutated sodium channels are trapped in an inactivated state.

### GENOTYPE-PHENOTYPE CORRELATIONS

Genotype-phenotype correlations match symptoms and response to treatment to gene mutation. This is done by carefully documenting the symptoms and response to treatment of patients who have had their mutation identified. Eventually this may allow the identification of genetic mutations by carefully looking at a patient's history and symptoms, and by comparing them to the histories and symptoms of those whose genetic mutation has been identified.

## AChR Remodeling

To understand the different types of CMS, we need to look at how the AChR is modeled, and remodeled, in the days following birth. The adult neuromuscular junction AChR is made up of five subunits. There are two alpha subunits, one beta, one delta, and one epsilon. Before birth there is a gamma subunit where the epsilon subunit will be in the mature NMJ.

During the first two weeks of life the NMJ undergoes remodeling, and the gamma subunit is replaced by an epsilon subunit. This remodeling is stimulated and coordinated by the nerve (axon) terminal and a protein called *acetylcholine receptor inducing activity* (ARIA). ARIA is found on the axon terminal and increases AchR activity tenfold.

The reasons for the remodeling of the NMJ are not clear, but animals whose NMJs do not make this switch die of impaired neuromuscular transmission, progressive muscle weakness and muscle atrophy within a few months of birth.

## Movement is Essential to Fetal Development

If a fetus doesn't move around normally as it is developing in the womb it may be born with inflexible arms and legs which are drawn close to the body. This condition is called *arthrogryposis multiplex congenita*. The CMS are just one cause of this condition.

Many CMS are caused by mutations of the epsilon subunit of the AChR, therefore problems do not arise until the NMJ remodeling begins, at birth or shortly thereafter. However, if the mutation affects one of the other subunits symptoms may begin while the child is still developing in the womb, and the baby may be born with arthrogryposis multiplex congenita.

## PRESYNAPTIC DEFECTS

The first group of congenital myasthenic syndromes we will look at are those which affect the presynaptic or nerve terminal side of the neuromuscular junction. These forms of CMS are caused by defects in ACh release, or in the ACh recycling process. It's estimated that presynaptic defects account for seven to eight percent of CMS cases.

### CHOLINE ACETYL-TRANSFERASE MYASTHENIA OR CHAT - CONGENITAL MG WITH EPISODIC APNEA

**INHERITANCE:** Recessive

**MUTATION:** The mutation responsible for the CMS known as *Choline-Acetyl Transferase Myasthenia* (ChAT) or *Familial Infantile Myasthenia* (FIM) is located on chromosome 10q11. ChAT is caused by a defect in the packaging or recycling process of ACh at the nerve terminal. In ChAT, endplate potentials (EPPs) are normal in the resting state, but decrease abnormally after stimulation. They then recover over 10 - 15 minutes.

**CLINICAL FEATURES:** ChAT is distinguished by sudden episodes of severe respiratory distress triggered by infection, fever, excitement, vomiting or too much physical activity. The symptoms of ChAT can begin before birth.

In one case a pregnant woman noticed that her developing baby was moving less than her previous babies had done during pregnancy. An ultrasound revealed that the baby had clenched fists and an unusually large amount of fluid in the uterus. (In some forms of CMS, fluid can build up in the uterus because the fetus is not swallowing as often or as strongly it should.)

At birth the infant girl had rigid hands and a lack of muscle tone. At 13 months she had episodes of apnea[41] brought on by an upper respiratory infection. She responded well to Mestinon®. Her older brother had died at the age of 15 hours from respiratory failure. He also had arthrogryposis,[42] which led physicians involved in his sister's care to conclude that he had also probably been affected by ChAT.

ChAT symptoms are often evident at birth or shortly thereafter, though sometimes symptoms don't become apparent until later. Babies with ChAT lack muscle tone, have ptosis of the eyelids which may come and go, have feeding difficulties and severe breathing problems.

---

41 Apnea: A temporary pause in breathing.
42 Arthrogryposis: The fixation of a joint in an extended or flexed position.

Crisis can be triggered in ChAT patients very rapidly by an infection, excitement, or vigorous play. The child may stop breathing during such a crisis and suffer brain injury or die due to a lack of oxygen.

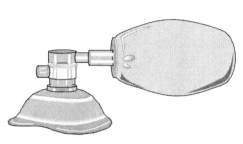

Parents and other caretakers should be trained in infant cardio-pulmonary resuscitation. Any infant with ChAT should sleep on an apnea monitor and parents should have an ambu-bag in the home. This device has a tight-fitting plastic mask which goes over the mouth and nose. The mask is connected to a bag which is squeezed by hand to force air into the lungs, and then relaxed to allow for exhalation. An ambu-bag allows a parent or caregiver to provide breathing support until medical help can be obtained. Medical supply houses should be able to fill your physician's prescription for an ambu-bag.

Between crises ChAT patients may have normal strength, or have mild myasthenic symptoms along with ptosis and a tendency to tire quickly. ChAT symptoms often gradually improve with age.

**TREATMENT:** ChAT is treated with anticholinesterase drugs such as Mestinon® and Prostigmine®.

### PAUCITY OF SYNAPTIC VESICLES AND REDUCED QUANTAL RELEASE:

**METHOD OF INHERITANCE:** Unknown;

This form of CMS is probably a result of a reduced number of synaptic vesicles at the axon (nerve) terminal. This reduction of vesicles is a result of a slow vesicle recycling rate, or slow transport of immature vesicles to the axon terminal. There can be more than an 80% reduction in the number of vesicles which produce, store and release ACh, so there's a marked reduction in the amount (quanta) of ACh released when the nerve is stimulated.

**CLINICAL FEATURES:** Symptoms start in infancy. Fatigability may be noted in face and limbs. The baby may have difficulty nursing, swallowing, crying and breathing. Some patients have variable ptosis and limitation of eye movements.

**TREATMENT:** AChE inhibitors like Mestinon®.

## REDUCED QUANTAL RELEASE BY NERVE TERMINALS

**METHOD OF INHERITANCE:** Unknown

**MUTATION:** Unknown

Only three patients with this form of presynaptic CMS have been described in medical literature. Studies revealed that there was a reduction of the action potential-dependent release of ACh while the spontaneous release of ACh remained normal. The result was a marked reduction in endplate potentials (EPPs), while miniature endplate potentials (MEPPs) were normal. Researchers found a structural flaw in the sac surrounding the vesicle, and theorize that the symptoms arise from an abnormal calcium release mechanism or impaired recycling of synaptic vesicles.

**CLINICAL FEATURES:** Onset is from birth to five years. Symptoms include weakness, difficulty coordinating limb and trunk movements, and nystagmus[43].

**TREATMENT:** In reported patients there was some improvement with a combination therapy of Mestinon® and 3,4 - Diaminopyridine (DAP).

## CONGENITAL LAMBERT-EATON MYASTHENIC SYNDROME (CLEMS)

**METHOD OF INHERITANCE:** Unknown.

In the autoimmune form of Lambert-Eaton Syndrome the immune system attacks one or more subunits in the calcium channels that trigger the release of ACh from the vesicle. The release of ACh is impaired not only at the NMJ but also at the junctions of autonomic nerves and other tissues, leading to symptoms which reach beyond muscle weakness. CLEMS' symptoms resemble those of autoimmune LEMS.

**MUTATION:** Unknown. The genes which control the ion subunits affected by the immune-system attack in Lambert-Eaton Myasthenic Syndrome (See LEMS - Chapter Four) are not mutated in CLEMS.

**CLINICAL FEATURES:** Onset is at birth. Only a few patients have been reported. Those described have had limb weakness, with feeding and swallowing problems.

A four-year-old child with CLEMS was reported to have had poor muscle tone and no reflexes since birth. Motor milestones

---

43 Nystagmus: involuntary, rhythmic movement of the eye, side-to-side, up and down, around or mixed.

(rolling over, sitting, walking etc.) were delayed. There were breathing and swallowing difficulties and limb weakness, as well as developmental delay. As is typical with LEMS, patients with CLEMS experience a brief increase in strength when they first exercise, but with sustained exercise they grow weak.

**TREATMENT:** Test results (EMG) improve when the patients are given DAP but the medication does little to relieve symptoms.

## SYNAPTIC BASAL LAMINA DEFECTS

### ENDPLATE AChE DEFICIENCY

**METHOD OF INHERITANCE:** Recessive or sporadic[44];
**MUTATION:** Chromosome 3P25

Endplate AChE deficiency was first reported in a single case in 1977, but more recently the characteristics of additional groups of patients have been described, giving a more complete understanding of this form of CMS. These mutations change the structure of the neuromuscular junction in the following ways:

- Reduce the size of the presynaptic axon terminals, which leads to a low number of quanta of ACh available for release, and a small number of EPPs.
- Lead to an absence of AChE secreted at the NMJ.
- Schwann cells[45] extend into the synaptic cleft.
- Simplified post-synaptic folds at some NMJs, so there's not room for adequate numbers of AChRs.

In one group all the patients had generalized weakness increased by exertion since birth. Eye movements were limited some of the time. All had a mild slowing of the reaction of the pupils of the eye to light. No patient in this group had Anti-AChR antibodies, but all had decremental EMG response typical of myasthenia. None responded to anticholinesterase medications, and anticholinesterases worsened symptoms in some patients. One of the patients had two siblings[46] who had died in early childhood of myasthenic symptoms; the other patients had no relatives with myasthenic symptoms.

---

44  Sporadic: A spontaneous genetic mutation. A genetic defect which is not inherited, but which can be passed on to the affected person's children.

45  Schwann cells: Specialized non-conducting cells that form the insulating covering (myelin sheath) of many axons.

46 Siblings: Brothers or sisters

Muscle studies from these patients revealed an absence of endplate acetylcholinesterase (EP AChE), prolonged endplate currents which were unaffected by cholinesterase inhibitors, a reduction in the amount of ACh (quantal release) when stimulated by nerve impulse and small presynaptic axon nerve endings.

Other studies revealed variations of the form, and suggest that modifying genes or environmental factors can partially compensate for the EP AChE deficiency.

**CLINICAL FEATURES:** There are several variants:

**VARIANT ONE:** Onset is birth to two years. The child reaches motor milestones later than average. Weakness is generalized. In some patients there is respiratory failure, reduced tendon reflexes, limitation of eye movements and pupils which are slow to respond to light. Exercise increases weakness. Older patients may develop scoliosis. Symptoms may progress, stabilize or improve over time, but this form of CMS is usually severely disabling.

**VARIANT TWO:** Partial AChE deficiency: Onset is before age six. Weakness is milder but progressive and can become disabling during the 20s.

**VARIANT THREE:** Mild symptoms in childhood. Symptoms worsen in the 50s, when patients can develop respiratory failure.

**TREATMENT:** There is none. Since AChE is lacking at the NMJ, giving an anticholinesterase drug like Mestinon® has no effect, or may worsen the weakness, since there's no AChE to oppose.

## POSTSYNAPTIC DEFECTS - AChR DISORDERS

## SLOW CHANNEL SYNDROMES

**METHOD OF INHERITANCE:** Autosomal Dominant;
**MUTATIONS:** AChR alpha subunit; Chromosome 2q24-q32;
AChR beta subunit; Chromosome 17p13.1;
AChR gamma subunit; Chromosome 2q33-q34;
Autosomal Dominant or Autosomal Recessive
AChR epsilon subunit; Chromosome 17p13-p12;

These mutations cause ACh to bind abnormally to the receptor site so that the ion channel opens repeatedly, does not fully shut or sticks in the open position. This causes an increased response to ACh. Thus a single nerve stimulus produces more than one action potential, sort of like a stutter. An ion channel that normally allows only sodium ions to enter the muscle sticks open long enough to allow unwanted calcium ions to also enter the muscle. This disrupts muscle contraction and damages the muscle cells. This damage accumulates over time, which explains why weakness progresses and symptoms grow worse as patients grow older.

Another cause of progressive weakness may be that the prolonged endplate potentials eventually "burn out" or depolarize the endplate which leads to failure of neuromuscular transmission. No one has yet explained why certain muscle groups are affected more than others and why symptoms vary so much from patient to patient.

**CLINICAL FEATURES:** Symptoms and severity of the slow channel syndromes vary from type to type. Unlike other CMS, in which the onset is during infancy or early childhood, the age of onset of the slow channel syndromes can be any time from birth to the 70s. Onset in women is commonly during pregnancy. Symptoms tend to be more severe when onset is early and milder when onset is later.

Symptoms include fatigability, ptosis and limitation of eye movements. In more severe cases there is facial weakness, weak eye closure, weakness and wasting of neck, shoulder, hand and finger muscles, scoliosis, weak legs, arms and respiratory muscles. Some patients have difficulties chewing and swallowing.

**TREATMENT:** AChE inhibitors either don't help or make symptoms worse. Quinidine Sulfate (200 mg. three - four times a day) is used to treat the slow channel syndromes. Quinidine has some potentially serious side effects including irregular heart rhythms, low blood pressure, ringing in the ears, headache, visual, hearing and digestive problems, as well as potential for allergic reaction. Patients with CMS occasionally grow worse and develop respiratory failure when given Quinidine. This possibility must be considered when starting the drug.

Recently, the drug fluoxetine (Prozac®) has been reported to relieve symptoms in slow channel syndrome. Dosage ranges from 80 - 100 mg. daily. Fluoxetine both blocks AChRs and increases the rate at which they close after releasing the ACh molecule. This appears to interrupt the "stuttering" process and stops the inappropriate flow of calcium into the muscle through sodium channels.

## FAST CHANNEL SYNDROMES

### AChR DEFICIENCY AND SHORT CHANNEL OPEN TIME

**METHOD OF INHERITANCE:** Autosomal Recessive;

In the fast channel syndromes there is a reduced response to ACh. These mutations affect the structure of the AChR site by causing the loss of an essential epsilon subunit. Without the epsilon subunit the ion channel will not function. To compensate, a gamma subunit is maintained where the epsilon subunit would normally be. This has several effects. It slows the opening of the channel and causes the channel to close more rapidly than it should. The post-synaptic fold is simplified, and there are fewer NMJs. The NMJs which do become established are longer than they should be.

**CLINICAL FEATURES:** Onset in reported cases has been before the age of two years. Weakness is generalized, including facial muscles, ptosis and limitation of eye movements. Severity varies; symptoms are non-progressive but persist into adulthood.

**TREATMENT:** AChE Inhibitors and DAP.

## ABNORMAL ACh-AChR INTERACTION:

### FAST-CHANNEL SYNDROMES DUE TO GATING ABNORMALITY

**METHOD OF INHERITANCE:** Autosomal Recessive;

These fast channel syndrome mutations cause a loss of function and abnormal ACh-AChR interaction. An open acetylcholine receptor site attracts ACh molecules. When ACh is released from the nerve terminal it heads for the nearest open receptor site. Acetylcholine binds to the channel, which then opens, and then closes again, with the ACh still bound. The ACh is then released to be recycled. The timing of the release is critical to the control of the channel's gating mechanism.

One of these mutations makes the AChR less attractive in the open state, so ACh is less likely to bind to the receptor site. Channel opening time is also slowed. The second fast channel gating mutation reduces the attractiveness of the AChR to ACh in the closed state. There are enough AChR sites, and the structure of the neuromuscular junctions and post synaptic folds are normal, but the AChR channels open fewer times and for a shorter interval than they should. This impairs the channel's gating efficiency.

**CLINICAL FEATURES:** In this form there are moderately severe myasthenic symptoms with generalized weakness. Onset is during infancy.

**TREATMENT:** DAP and perhaps Mestinon®.

## FAST CHANNEL SYNDROME WITH ARTHROGRYPOSIS MULTIPLEX CONGENITA:

**METHOD OF INHERITANCE:** Autosomal Recessive;

This form of CMS is caused by mutations in the delta subunit of the AChR. These mutations begin to affect the function of the muscle earlier than epsilon subunit mutations which do not usually affect a child until after birth. In this form of CMS the ion channel responds to stimulation for too short a period of time, and the current generated ends too quickly. This malfunction affects both fetal and adult AChRs.

When a fetus doesn't move around as it should while it is developing in the womb it may be born with a condition called arthrogryposis multiplex congenita, in which the arms and legs are drawn up against the body and cannot be straightened.

In one reported case, a mother noted that the child she was carrying, her fourth, did not move as much as her previous healthy children had done during development. The little girl was born with clenched fists and experienced breathing problems on the day of birth. She was described as floppy, with a weak cry. She would choke while feeding. Over the first few months of life she had severe breathing problems and required respiratory support on occasion.

The baby girl was admitted to hospital at the age of four months and diagnosed with CMS. Treatment with Mestinon® was begun. She responded well to treatment and began walking at 14 months. At six years her symptoms include fatigable weakness of arms and legs limiting her ability to walk distances of more than a block or to climb many stairs. She had fatigable ptosis, limitation of eye movements and occasional swallowing problems.

**CLINICAL FEATURES:** In this form of CMS the mother may notice that the growing baby does not move as much in the womb as babies in previous pregnancies. An ultrasound exam may reveal that the baby has rigid or abnormally flexed joints. At birth the infant may have clenched fists, or inflexible limbs drawn up to the body. There is generalized weakness, including limbs, limitation of eye movements, difficulty nursing and swallowing and respiratory failure.

**TREATMENT:** AChE inhibitors such as Mestinon®.

## REDUCED EXPRESSION OF ACHRS AND SEVERE WEAKNESS

**METHOD OF INHERITANCE:** Autosomal Recessive;

This mutation causes major disruptions in both the structure and function of the neuromuscular junction. It interrupts the normal interaction between the beta and delta subunits. It also affects the assembly of the five subunits so that they form an abnormal AChR, which doesn't work as it should. The affected NMJs don't imbed themselves into the muscle membrane as they do normally, but remain inside the cytoplasm of the cell, where they can't do any work. Fewer than 10% of the NMJs function as they should.

**CLINICAL FEATURES:** Onset is at birth with generalized severe weakness and respiratory failure. There is difficulty with nursing and swallowing. The child needs respiratory support to survive, but the weakness does not progress.

**TREATMENT:** There is some response to Mestinon®.

## DELTA SUBUNIT MUTATIONS WITH REDUCED EXPRESSION OF ACHRS AND FAST CHANNEL EFFECTS

**METHOD OF INHERITANCE:** Recessive;

In this form of CMS there is a reduction in the number of AChRs at the NMJ. The delta and alpha subunits do not assemble properly during AChR formation. The ion channels in the NMJ open too slowly, close too quickly and do not attract ACh normally. ACh leaves the binding site on the AChR too quickly. Some endplates have reduced or shallow junctional folds. Endplate current is weak and doesn't last long enough to produce strong muscle contractions.

**CLINICAL FEATURES:** So far this form has been found only in a small group of Saudi Arabian patients. Onset is from birth. An affected infant has reduced muscle tone, generalized severe weakness and severe breathing difficulties, sometimes even respiratory failure. Patients have facial weakness including limitation of eye movements and ptosis. Neck muscles are very weak, limb muscles only moderately so. Affected infants have difficulties sucking and swallowing, and later have problems with speech. Weakness tends to diminish with age. Patients are small in stature with large ears, a small jaw and a high, arched palate.

**TREATMENT:** There is some response to Mestinon® in combination with DAP.

## RAPSYN MUTATIONS

### REDUCED EXPRESSION OF AChRS

**METHOD OF INHERITANCE:** Recessive

**MUTATION:** Rapsyn; Chromosome 11p11.2-p11.1

Rapsyn plays a vital role in the formation of AChRs. Rapsyn molecules cluster, attach to the endplate membrane and send out a signal that attracts AChRs, which they bind to the membrane. Rapsyn mutations reduce rapsyn's ability to bind AChRs to the endplate. This causes a reduction in AChRs to 10 - 48% of normal.

**CLINICAL FEATURES:** Onset may be before birth. The mother may notice reduced fetal movements. The baby may be born with limbs which are drawn up and inflexible. Some patients develop symptoms shortly after birth or during infancy, though a few patients don't develop symptoms until adulthood.

Symptoms vary in severity even between patients who have the same mutation. Infants have reduced muscle tone, a weak cry, respiratory failure, difficulty nursing and ptosis. Symptoms worsen when the patient has an infection and fever. Affected children often walk in their second year but continue to experience generalized weakness and fatigue. Ptosis continues but there is no limitation of eye movements. Weak jaw muscles may lead to chewing problems. The small jaw caused by this mutation can lead to misaligned and crowded teeth.

**TREATMENT:** Some response to Mestinon® and DAP.

### RAPSYN MUTATION WITH FACIAL MALFORMATIONS

**METHOD OF INHERITANCE:** Recessive;

**MUTATION:** Rapsyn ; Chromosome 11p11.2-p11.1;

This form has been reported in only one group of Jewish patients from 10 families of Iraqi or Iranian origins believed to have had a common ancestor.

**CLINICAL FEATURES:** Onset is in infancy. The facial changes seen in this form of CMS are obvious by age two. Affected children develop a long, narrow face with protruding jaws, badly misaligned teeth and a high-arched palate. Muscle weakness is restricted mostly to the face. There is ptosis and tiring when speaking or chewing. Symptoms are mild and weakness does not progress though the appearance is quite affected.

**TREATMENT:** Mestinon®

## FAMILIAL LIMB-GIRDLE MYASTHENIA

**METHOD OF INHERITANCE:** Autosomal recessive or sporadic[47];

**CLINICAL FEATURES:** Onset for the inherited (recessive) form can be from infancy to the teens. Onset for the sporadic form can be from the teens to the 40s. Onset for women is typically during a pregnancy.

Limb-girdle CMS affects the muscles around both hips and both shoulders with weakness, fatigue, muscle wasting, cramps and muscle pain. Symptoms are slowly progressive. Muscles may become contracted. Some patients have a heart rhythm defect. Weakness is made worse by exercise.

One study reported two sisters with limb-girdle CMS. The 22-year-old complained of severe weakness in her hip girdle and knees after walking for ten minutes and weakness in her legs after climbing two to three flights of stairs. Her jaw tired with prolonged chewing. Her symptoms began at the age of four years.

She had never had breathing problems, double vision or ptosis. Her muscles seemed normal at rest. Muscle tone was normal. There was no noticeable fatigability involving the eye, throat, facial or tongue muscles. Routine blood work and a muscle biopsy revealed no abnormalities. The acetylcholine receptor antibody test was negative. Nerve conduction studies and needle EMG were normal at rest, but after the patient climbed a flight of stairs three times in quick succession, the EMG showed significant decrement in some of her leg muscles.

Her strength improved dramatically with IV administration of 10 mg of Tensilon®, leading to a diagnosis of limb-girdle myasthenia. She was prescribed 30 mg. of Mestinon® three times a day. After two weeks on Mestinon® she was able to climb a flight of stairs seven times before becoming weak.

Her younger sister, 18 years old, had almost the same symptoms and test results. Her EMG, which was normal at rest, also showed decremental response following strenuous exercise. She had a similar response to Tensilon and responded well to Mestinon® therapy.

**Treatment:** Mestinon® and DAP.

---

47 Sporadic: Caused by a spontaneous mutation which is not inherited.

## MuSK MUTATIONS: REDUCED EXPRESSION OF AChRs

**METHOD OF INHERITANCE:** Recessive;

**MUTATION:** MuSK; Chromosome 9q31.3-q32;

**CLINICAL FEATURES:** Symptoms begin during infancy and include breathing difficulties, chewing and swallowing problems, fatigue, ptosis, weakness (worse in arms than in legs, and worse in muscles close to the body, like shoulders and neck). Symptoms improve with age, but may become worse during pregnancy.

**TREATMENT:** DAP, no benefit from Mestinon®.

## SODIUM CHANNEL MUTATION

This disorder has been described in only one patient. It combines features of CMS and another inherited neuromuscular disorder, Periodic Paralysis. Several forms of Periodic Paralysis are caused by mutations in the sodium channel, and it's possible that this particular CMS may eventually be reclassified as a Periodic Paralysis.

### WEAKNESS+ EPISODIC APNEA & BULBAR DYSFUNCTION

**METHOD OF INHERITANCE:** Dominant;

**MUTATION:** Sodium Channel - alpha subunit (SCN4A); Chromosome 17q35;

This mutation causes the voltage-gated sodium ion channel to inactivate too quickly. As a result the action potential is not passed on to the muscle.

**CLINICAL FEATURES:** Only one patient has been described. From birth she has had from one to three abrupt attacks of paralysis monthly lasting from three to thirty minutes. During attacks her muscles are completely flaccid and she becomes unable to breathe. She reached motor milestones late, tires easily and has ptosis. She has facial, trunk and limb weakness, worsened by activity. She can only walk a short distance and hold her arms horizontally for only 20 seconds. She is developmentally delayed, probably the result of oxygen deprivation during episodes of respiratory failure.

**TREATMENT:** Mestinon® and acetazolamide (Diamox®), a carbonic anhydrase inhibitor. Carbonic anhydrase inhibitors are used to treat some sodium channel disorders which cause Periodic Paralysis.

## Notes:

# 7

# WHAT ABOUT OUR CHILDREN?

Patients who have the acquired (autoimmune) form of MG sometimes worry that they may pass the disease on to their children or grandchildren. Very occasionally autoimmune MG occurs in more than one member of a family, leading to medical speculation that, perhaps, there is an element of inheritance involved. This has not been an easy question to answer in the past, but the more sophisticated diagnostic and genetic tools now available make the answer to this question more clear.

## CAN ACQUIRED MG BE INHERITED?

Many studies have been conducted in an attempt to determine if autoimmune MG occurs, in a mild, unrecognized form, in relatives of diagnosed MG patients. As of yet none of these studies have shown that idiopathic MG is directly inherited. In the general population MG occurs in one person in 7,000 - 10,000. The proportion of cases among those that have a close relative with autoimmune MG is estimated to be between 1.2 and 4.3%.

In the most convincing case of familial autoimmune MG, a family was described in which the parents were first cousins. Five of their 10 children developed MG, with age of onset ranging from 50 - 72 years. Three of them had elevated anti-AChR antibodies. The researchers excluded all the known genetic mutations as a cause for their MG but suggested that a genetic predisposition was a factor.

Since the parents of these patients were first cousins both may have carried an inherited predisposition to be vulnerable to MG under the right circumstances. This predisposition, multiplied by two, may have been inherited by some of their children who developed MG when exposed to the right triggering factors.

Certainly, if there is genetic predisposition to develop MG it is *only* a predisposition. Perhaps the slightly higher rate of MG among identical twins is due to sharing both the same genetic predisposition and the same early environment. No one can say with absolute certainty. In the meantime, patients can take comfort from the knowledge that autoimmune MG is *not* a hereditary disease and their children and grandchildren are in little danger of developing it.

## PREGNANCY AND MYASTHENIA

Young women who have MG are usually concerned about the effect the disease will have on their ability to bear children. It is impossible to predict how a specific patient will respond to the physical and hormonal stresses of pregnancy and birth. However, most myasthenic women have quite successful pregnancies and deliveries.

The best course of action for an affected woman contemplating pregnancy is to seek counseling beforehand. It may rarely be necessary to reduce or discontinue medications known to be toxic to a developing child. Also, the physiological changes the body undergoes during pregnancy require ongoing and careful management, as many women find themselves more symptomatic during the early months of pregnancy.

Studies have shown that in about one in three myasthenic women symptoms improve during pregnancy. A third find their symptoms unaffected. The remaining third find their symptoms become worse. Oddly enough, a woman may find that this pattern of improvement or worsening symptoms varies from pregnancy to pregnancy. Many women report that symptoms are worse during the earlier stages of pregnancy, but that they feel better as the pregnancy progresses. It is common for women to have less weakness than usual in the last trimester of pregnancy. Worsening of symptoms is more common during the first few months after delivery, when it can be managed with the usual treatments.

## DRUGS AND PREGNANCY

Myasthenia gravis is treated with powerful drugs, and it's only natural that a myasthenic woman carrying a child might be concerned about their effects on her growing baby. The question of whether to discontinue one's medications is not to be taken lightly.

## THE ANTICHOLINESTERASES

There have been no reports of harmful effects to infants born to myasthenic women who were being treated with the anticholinesterase drugs, Mestinon®, Prostigmine® and Mytelase®. These drugs cross the placental barrier, so they reach the fetus in about the same concentration as that found in the mother's blood. It has been suggested that the onset of neonatal MG might be delayed in affected infants due to anticholinesterases in the baby's blood at birth.

## STEROIDS

There is no evidence that taking steroids in usual doses during pregnancy has any ill effect on a developing fetus, but large doses (over 50 mg.) may increase the risk of having a large baby or developing *gestational diabetes*[48].

## AZATHIOPRINE

Imuran® (azathioprine), should not be taken during pregnancy (or at any other time) without carefully weighing the risks versus the benefits, but if a woman needs azathioprine to control her symptoms, and becomes pregnant there is little evidence that it is necessary to discontinue the medication.

There is no new data available on women with MG treated with azathioprine who have given birth, but there are a few new studies following women with other immune-system disorders who were treated with azathioprine, or its active metabolite[49], 6- mercaptopurine (6 - MP). These studies are useful in the absence of studies specific to MG.

One study followed 155 pregnancies in patients with inflammatory bowel disease (including men who fathered children) while taking 6-MP. There was no increase in miscarriage, spontaneous abortion due to birth defect, major birth defects, cancer or increased rate of infections among male or female patients taking 6MP compared with others not taking the drug. The conclusion was that the drug was safe for use during pregnancy. While there are some risks to taking azathioprine during a pregnancy, it may be necessary to

---

48 Gestational diabetes: A form of diabetes which begins during pregnancy in women who have not been known to have diabetes before, and usually disappears following delivery.

49 Metabolite: A substance produced by metabolism.

preserve strength and life. When that is the case, the weight of medical evidence is reasonably reassuring that major harm is not done.

## PLASMA EXCHANGE AND IVIG

Plasma exchange and IVIG may be as safely performed during pregnancy as at any other time and do not harm the developing infant. Plasma exchange or IVIG of the mother is used at times to treat affected infants while they are still in the uterus (in utero).

## BIRTH

Studies show that women with MG have a slightly increased rate of medical intervention during delivery. This may be linked to anxiety about delivery in MG.

One study reviewed all births occurring in Norway from 1967 through 2000, using data from the Medical Birth Registry of Norway. This study compared 127 births by mothers with MG to births to women without MG. It found that women with MG had a slightly higher rate of complications at delivery (40.9% vs 32.9%).

In particular, the risk of pre-term rupture of amniotic membranes was three times higher in the MG group compared to the reference group (5.5% vs 1.7%). The rate of interventions during birth was raised (33.9% vs 20.0%) and the number of cesarean sections doubled (17.3% vs 8.6%).

Another study followed 12 women, ages 25 - 36, through 12 pregnancies in which they delivered 14 children. One women delivered twice, and there was one twin pregnancy. Clinical symptoms of myasthenia worsened in five women. One was admitted twice to the intensive care unit during her pregnancy. Two were admitted to intensive care unit during the first month after their baby's birth.

The pregnancies lasted an average 39.3 weeks (ranged from 38 – 40.6 weeks), so none of the women with MG delivered significantly pre-term. All birth weights were normal: 3329 grams (2660 – 4520 grams). Six women delivered vaginally, two by instrumental extraction and five by cesarean section. Apgar score[50] was normal for all infants: 9/10. Three of the infants developed neonatal myasthenia. It was recommended that obstetrical monitoring in a well-equipped

---

50 Apgar score: A test done one minute and five minutes after birth to determine a newborn baby's physical health. Scoring is based on five factors that rate how well a baby is adjusting to life outside the womb.

medical center be the standard of care for pregnant women with MG because of the risk of neonatal myasthenia. For safety, observation of both mother and infant are necessary for several days after the birth.

## ANESTHESIAS

Epidural anesthesia is currently the agent of choice for decreasing pain during labor. Forceps or vacuum delivery will shorten the second stage of labor in patients who are unable to push repetitively or forcefully enough. Narcotic and sedative medications may be used in the presence of careful, continuous, assessment but they may increase MG symptoms.

The uterus itself is composed of smooth (involuntary) muscle and is not affected by MG. During the first stage of labor, when only the uterus is involved, there is little or no difference between the myasthenic woman's labor and the unaffected woman's labor. But during the second stage of labor the baby must be pushed from the mother's body by muscular effort. This stage may be slowed if the mother is weak and fatigues easily. This rarely prevents a mother from delivering vaginally, and on average the myasthenic woman's labor is no longer than that of other women.

Enemas have been reported to cause exacerbation of MG symptoms by some women. Many maternity units give an enema to laboring patients as part of their "prep". If this is a concern discuss it with your attending physician *beforehand.* A letter from the doctor which can be taken to the hospital stating how prep is to be done is good insurance. Prep is generally done very soon after the mother arrives at the hospital, before the attending physician is called. Anesthetics of choice should also be discussed and instructions left on the maternity floor in case the need arises for their use.

## BREAST FEEDING

Drugs taken by a nursing mother can pass into breast milk. The anticholinesterases have been reported to cause colic in some breast-fed newborns, but in no case have MG medications caused abnormalities in an infant who breast feeds. Anti-AChR antibodies secreted in the mother's milk do not pass to the infant in significant amounts, and any which the milk contains are digested along with the milk, not absorbed into the blood. Myasthenic mothers can safely breast feed their infants without fear of MG-related problems.

## HOME WITH THE BABY

The postpartum period is often associated with an increase in symptoms and a higher incidence of exacerbation. Common sense suggests that the new mother arrange for help with the baby and household responsibilities. Grandmothers, sisters, aunts, friends, even a paid aide can take some of the load off while things settle down.

Shopping for all the necessities a new baby needs should be done well in advance so that everything is in place before the big day. Try to keep the baby's everyday clothing simple. Choose Velcro® fasteners on clothing instead of ties, buttons and snaps.

A high-wheeled pram or baby buggy can save lots of lifting and carrying. A dressing table where you can bathe, change and dress the baby without bending over is a must. It should be equipped with rails and have a safety strap. *Never* assume your baby will not move about or roll over while you bend down to pick up a dropped object.

Take advantage of the baby's naps to get the rest you need. Dishes and ironing can wait. You need to conserve your strength. If you have family nearby they may be more willing than you realize to pitch in and give you a hand. Babies attract friends and neighbors in the nicest way. If the advice makes you feel defensive or inadequate, listen politely, thank the "advisee" and promptly forget what doesn't feel supportive or right. Just relax and let those you love help you.

If you're weepy, tired and out of sorts, you're in good company. Even perfectly healthy new mothers get the blues. It's partly exhaustion, partly apprehension and partly hormonal adjustment. Things will settle down in a few months. But stress and real depression can worsen MG symptoms. Treatment with Prednisone® can also cause or worsen insomnia, anxiety and depression.

If your new responsibilities threaten to overwhelm you shouldn't hesitate to seek your physician's help. Medication may need to be adjusted as your body returns to the pre-pregnant state. It's vitally important to do all you can to ease your passage through a potentially difficult but also very joyous and exciting time.

## VACCINATION PRECAUTIONS

As an infant approaches 12 weeks it is time to begin the vaccinations which will protect her from the childhood diseases that once claimed the lives of so many children. One of these vaccinations guards against the polio viruses. There are two types of polio vaccine available, one injectable, the other oral. The injectable vaccine consists of inactive polio virus, but the oral form contains weakened live virus. The child given oral polio vaccine will shed live polio virus in the stool for four to six weeks. These weakened viruses pose no threat normally, but anyone who has not been vaccinated previously and who is on immunosuppressant therapy may be at risk of contracting polio. If the infant's caretaker or other family members are on immunosuppressants the infant should be given the injectable form of the vaccine if at all possible.

## TRANSIENT NEONATAL MG

Most infants whose mothers have MG are perfectly healthy at birth, but 9 - 20% develop a temporary form of myasthenia called transient neonatal MG (NMG). This may happen even in women with no detectable antibodies, since maternal antibodies are able to cross the placenta and may affect the infant's AChRs.

Most infants with NMG appear normal at birth but develop weakness within a few hours. The child with NMG usually has problems nursing, swallowing and breathing. Diagnosis is made when Mestinon® or a similar drug relieves the weakness and allows the child to feed and breathe more normally. Infants born to myasthenic mothers require constant monitoring by an alert nursing staff for the first several days of life.

There is no test available to determine if an unborn infant will develop NMG after birth, but one strong indication that the baby is affected is a mother who develops polyhydramnios[51]. The volume of fluid in the uterus may increase because the baby has stopped swallowing. This increase in uterine fluid volume during the late stages of pregnancy is occasionally the first symptom of MG in the mother. It has been suggested that anti-AChR antibody testing should be considered in all cases of unexplained polyhydramnios. Babies who develop symptoms before birth are sometimes diagnosed by ultrasound after the mother notices that the child's movements have slowed.

Symptoms which develop while the baby is still in the womb may become life-threatening. It may be necessary to take steps to decrease the number of antibodies crossing from the mother to the fetus. Treatment may include starting or increasing steroids, or using plasma exchange.

---

51 Polyhydramnios: The presence of excessive amniotic fluid.

The risk to the baby's life from NMG is at its peak during the first week of life and then declines. Infants with NMG almost always recover completely by the age of 12 weeks, but may require medication and respiratory assistance in the meantime.

One report was of a young woman with MG whose first pregnancy was complicated during the third trimester by polyhydramnios. When the child was born it had generalized muscle weakness, respiratory distress, a weak cry, anemia and poor sucking ability. It was necessary to put the baby on a respirator. The diagnosis of NMG was confirmed with repetitive nerve stimulation which showed the decrement typical of MG, and by the presence of anti-AChR antibodies. The infant was treated with anticholinesterase for three months. After 26 days of hospitalization, the baby was released. Myasthenic symptoms eventually went away and there were no side effects of the treatment. A second pregnancy was normal and the second newborn was completely healthy.

There is no evidence to suggest that infants who have NMG are any more likely to develop autoimmune MG later in life than other children. In one long-term study 31 children of myasthenic mothers were followed for up to 31 years. Eleven of these children developed NMG at birth. All of them went on to become healthy. Twenty-nine of the 31 had no signs of neuromuscular disease, and none had anti-AChR antibodies Two of the children who had NMG had some myopathy[52], which the researchers felt was probably unrelated to the mother's MG.

## JUVENILE MG

Unfortunately, children do occasionally develop MG. In children the disorder is called juvenile myasthenia gravis (JMG), but it is essentially the same disease as adult acquired (autoimmune) MG. Juvenile MG is treated the same way as adult MG, taking into account the patient's age and the effect of drugs and treatment on growth.

There's no significant difference between the number of boys and girls who develop JMG. Younger children seem to develop ocular MG more frequently than do older ones. Ocular symptoms like ptosis (droopy eyelids) are often the first symptom, but many children go on to develop more generalized symptoms. Anti-AChR antibodies are detected more frequently among children with generalized disease than those with only ocular symptoms. The Tensilon® (edrophonium

---

52 Myopathy: muscle disease.

chloride) and Prostigmine® (neostigmine methylsulfate) tests are positive in the large majority of children with MG.

Several Thai clinicians wrote of their shared experience caring for patients with JMG. Together they had cared for 27 children with MG. In all cases, the diagnosis was confirmed by a combination of clinical examination and neostigmine test. Over 90% of their patients developed only ocular myasthenia to begin with. Average onset of symptoms was 33 months. About 24% of these patients went on to develop generalized weakness. (This is a lower percentage than in adults, where at least 66% of those who began with only ocular symptoms develop generalized MG.) A few patients (eight per cent) developed respiratory failure requiring respiratory support. Thymectomy was performed on 10 patients. Complete remissions were achieved in about 70% and partial remissions in 26% of cases with the combination of Imuran® and Mestinon®. None of the patients experienced a myasthenic crisis.

Another study followed 27 children with MG for a period of 25 years after they first developed symptoms and noted the following: Onset was after 10 years of age in the majority of patients. At onset half had only ocular symptoms, the other half had generalized weakness. Half of those with ocular-onset went on to develop generalized weakness. Sixty-three percent had anti-AChR antibodies (Ed Note: This was before MuSK antibodies were discovered). There was no difference between the number of girls and boys who were antibody-positive.

The majority of patients with only ocular myasthenia were treated with Mestinon®. As symptoms progressed other therapies were needed. All patients who were given corticosteroids ultimately underwent thymectomy.

As a rule, early-onset MG appears to have the same course as in adult life and responds to the same kinds of therapy. Children who have autoimmune MG (anti-AChR antibody type) generally respond well to thymectomy. Most neurologists recommend thymectomy for generalized MG in childhood, except in infants under the age of one year whose immune systems have yet to mature, and for whom such surgery might have long-term effects on immunological development. Immune suppressant therapy is effective with no major side-effects and should be considered in seriously affected children who do not respond to less aggressive therapies.

## THE CONGENITAL MYASTHENIC SYNDROMES

The congenital myasthenic syndromes (CMS) are a group of rare genetic disorders which affect neuromuscular transmission. The symptoms of the CMS are caused by genetic errors which cause malfunctions in one or more areas of the NMJ.

The congenital myasthenias cause muscle weakness and fatigability similar to those of autoimmune MG. The symptoms of CMS usually begin within the first two years of life, although some patients with Slow Channel Syndrome, Familial Limb-Girdle Myasthenia and some Rapsyn mutations have delayed onset. Patients with those forms have been reported to develop symptoms as late as in the 60s and 70s.

The symptoms of CMS vary from mild to severe. Weakness is limited to ocular and facial muscles in some forms, while in other forms the ability to breathe and swallow are affected and symptoms can become life-threatening. It's also possible for patients with the same form, even members of the same family, to be affected to differing degrees.

Diagnosis of CMS can be difficult. Patients with some forms of CMS may not respond to Tensilon®, or may worsen with its administration, and may not show the typical decremental responses on EMG and nerve conduction studies, especially if distal muscles (hands) are tested rather than proximal (facial, neck) muscles.

Patients with CMS are sometimes helped by medications that inhibit the breakdown of acetylcholine or increase its release. Some respond to quinine, others to 3,4 - Diaminopyridine (DAP). Thymectomy is of no benefit. Since the CM syndromes don't involve the immune system, medications and treatments that suppress the immune system aren't used. See Chapter Six, The Congenital Myasthenias; for an in-depth discussion of genetic factors, information on each of the various forms of CMS and specific treatments for each form.

## HEALTH CONSIDERATIONS

Parenting a child with myasthenia is a challenge. The common childhood fevers, chest congestion and viruses may pose a real danger, as they often make MG symptoms worse. The child with MG or a CMS should be kept away from other children who are ill, or suffering from colds or upper respiratory infections. Family, friends and the parents of playmates should be made aware of the danger of infection to your child. Teach your child to wash his hands thoroughly after using the toilet and before eating. Teach him to keep his fingers, toys and other objects out of his mouth.

## DIET

Encourage a varied diet, emphasizing whole foods over sweets and fast foods. Light meals with nutritious snacks in between may be easier for your child to manage than three large meals a day.

Fruit smoothies are an excellent light meal or snack which can be made in the blender. They are easy to swallow and attractive, even to picky eaters. Milk and cottage cheese, with frozen berries or other fruit, can be whipped up in a tasty combination which provides the nutrition necessary for growth.

### RECIPE FOR A FRUIT SMOOTHIE
*Put in the blender:*
¾ cup milk and ¾ cup 2% cottage cheese.
Blend until smooth.
*Add* ½ cup fresh or frozen unsweetened berries
(strawberries, blueberries etc.) or a fresh nectarine or
peach cut into pieces, and one small banana.
*Add* more milk as needed to keep mixture liquid enough
to blend. You should end up with four cups.
*Add* ½ tsp vitamin C powder or crush a 500 mg. vitamin
C tablet and add it, blending it in. The vitamin C keeps
the fruit from turning brown.
Three-quarters of a cup of smoothie makes an excellent
breakfast with a poached or soft boiled egg. A ½ cup
serving can be used as a mid-meal or bedtime snack.

## MEDICATION

When you have myasthenia, medication is one of the facts of life. There are small plastic pillboxes with compartments for individual doses of medication. Some of these have alarms that can be programmed to beep at a required time. These are especially useful when the child becomes responsible for taking her own medications. Organizing the day's medication ahead of time allows you to relax and not worry about missed doses.

Children over five or six who are physically able should be increasingly responsible for their own care. By the time children are ten or twelve they should be responsible for taking their own medications, under gentle supervision. They should be taught the effects of an overdose and understand the consequences of missing doses. It's often hard for parents to let go and allow a child to assume responsibility for their medications, but it's best to have this routine established before the child reaches adolescence. Teens can become rebellious about taking medication. Parents who insist on doling out and supervising the swallowing of every pill risk making medication a control issue with a teen. Parents need to learn to allow the child to have autonomy in this area. The resolve to let a teen take care of their own medication may be tested when the child forgets one or more doses, but resist the urge to step in. Teens want to keep up with peers, and that's great motivation for taking one's pills on schedule.

### THE SCHOOL-AGE CHILD AND MYASTHENIA

Myasthenia poses unique problems for school-age youngsters. A child's strength may vary widely from day-to-day, even from hour-to-hour, which is not just frustrating for teachers but is extremely difficult for the child. It is impossible to set out guidelines which will work for every child, or even which will work for one child every day. Some parents of chronically ill children complain that inflexibility of school staff is one of the biggest challenges they face. School staff sometimes don't understand the variations in strength children with chronic illnesses face, and are reluctant, or unwilling, to make allowances for a child with physical problems.

The school should be educated regarding the child's MG so that the child is evaluated fairly and expectations are kept reasonable. A medical alert bracelet or necklace should be worn at all times.

### ALLOW THE CHILD TO SET THE PACE

The child knows best how they feel. Sometimes an hour's rest in the nurse's office will allow the child to finish the school day, and can avoid the loss of an afternoon's classwork. School staff need to be flexible and allow children with chronic illnesses to adapt their activities to the current strength level.

## CLASSROOM MODIFICATIONS

There are many ways to support children so that their daily life at school is easier. Several issues to consider are: Intensity of activity, temperature control and adequate rest. The school must work with the parent to meet the needs of the individual child.

If classroom desks and equipment are stressing your child physically ask the school about consulting with an occupational therapist. The therapist can ensure proper desk and seat size and identify modifications which will help the child be comfortable. It is vital that the child be in a desk which does not stress weak muscle areas. If neck pain or weakness is a problem there is a device called a slant board, that attaches to the school desk. It can lie flat or be raised up at an angle, and makes writing or reading easier. Additional modifications may also be needed depending on the day, time of day, etc. For example, some children may need the help of a note-taker on days when they are not strong. This note-taking may be done by an aide or in the upper grades, by another student.

There should be a designated place in the classroom the child can go if they feel fatigued or weak. This might be a futon, a bean bag chair or a supportive rocking chair. Some children may require a rest period mid-day in order to complete the school day. This may mean a nap in the nurse's office, or quietly curling up in a large supportive chair or sofa in the classroom.

In schools where classrooms are on two or more levels arrangements may have to be made for the child to attend classes on the main floor. If the child changes classrooms they may need to leave class a few minutes early to have time to negotiate hallways and stairs safely, and they may need a friend to carry their books.

## GYM CLASS

By law, schools must accommodate children with disabilities. Period. Some children with myasthenia can be moderately active, some can be very active, but there are some who have very little tolerance for exercise. These children may experience crisis if they are pushed beyond their physical capacity.

Gym teachers must be made aware of the harmful effects of overheating and of the possibility of fluctuating strength levels. The child must be allowed to judge his own tolerance for activity in doubtful situations. Gym teachers should also be prepared to protect the myasthenic child who may not want to quit before his or her peers. The urge to keep up physically is strong, and some kids will push themselves unwisely unless guided by a knowing adult.

## WHO'S ON YOUR TEAM?

In most cases school staff and teachers are a caring team which works to make the educational experience a positive one for the myasthenic child. A parent may occasionally need the support of the child's pediatrician or neurologist to impress upon the school just how important it is to adapt the child's environment and routine to his strength levels. Don't hesitate to call in your child's physician if needed.

Lastly, the child with MG should be allowed to *be a child*, and not be placed under undue restrictions by parents who are afraid of infections or accidents. The child with MG should also be expected to work to capacity and not be allowed to take refuge in their disability. It should also be recognized that at times it may be difficult for the child to cope successfully with the challenges they face. No one, child or adult, copes well all the time. Allowances have to be made for those times when it gets to be too much.

Parents will feel the strain. Anxiety, guilt, (Is this my fault?) fear and anger may color attitudes and events on a day - to - day basis. Parents shouldn't expect perfection from their child *or* themselves. Parenting is a big job with a healthy child, let alone one with a chronic medical problem. It's easier if everyone maintains a sense of humor.

Children learn how to deal with their MG from those around them, and it is best treated with a matter-of-fact attitude. It's a problem, but not an insurmountable one. Illness isn't anyone's fault, and blaming uses up energy which could be used elsewhere. Myasthenia doesn't limit the amount of love a person can give or receive and, love not illness, should be the foundation of  familial relationships.

# 8

# CRISIS

The term *crisis* is used when an MG patient becomes unable to breathe adequately, or the swallowing capacity is so compromised that the patient chokes on his own saliva and can neither eat or drink. Crisis may result from taking too little anticholinesterase or immunosuppressant medication or (very rarely) from taking too much. It may also be caused by an infection, trauma, stress or some other underlying medical problem.

## CRISIS PROCEDURES

Although procedures vary, the myasthenic who is in crisis will often be admitted to the intensive care unit. They will sometimes be put on a ventilator, receive food and fluids through a nasal-gastric feeding tube[53.] They may be taken off their anticholinesterase medication or have the dosage reduced. This allows the patient to rest for 48 hours.

Any infection or other medical condition will be treated while the patient is resting. The supervision of a neurologist is vital, as it may be necessary to start plasma exchange (PE) or intravenous immunoglobulin (IVIG) treatments and begin, or adjust, treatment with immunosuppressants.

Crisis was once a truly life-threatening state, but it is now much less so, due to technology and therapeutic advances. Patients can usually be stabilized within hours or days, but still need reassurance and a great deal of support during this difficult time.

If a myasthenic has significant breathing difficulties, or has experienced respiratory crisis in the past, it can be reassuring to have an ambu-bag on hand at home and when traveling. This device is

---

53 Nasal-gastric feeding tube: A flexible feeding tube which is inserted through the nose, down the throat and into the stomach.

often used in ambulances and
hospital emergency rooms. It
has a tight fitting plastic mask
which goes over the mouth and
nose. The mask is connected to
a bag which is squeezed by
hand to force air into the lungs
and then relaxed to allow for
exhalation. If a patient becomes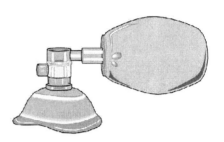
unable to breathe adequately a friend or family member can use the
ambu-bag to maintain respiration until help has arrived or the patient
is taken to a hospital. Medical supply houses should be able to fill
your physician's prescription for an ambu-bag.

## HOSPITAL CARE FOR OTHER CONDITIONS

Medical staff involved in caring for a myasthenic hospitalized for
reasons other than myasthenia need to be aware that crisis can be
induced in a previously stabilized patient by surgery, trauma (an auto
accident, burns, falls, etc.), infections or other medications. It is
important that the nursing staff be alert to early symptoms of
deterioration in MG patients.

Some hospitals will leave a patient's anticholinesterases at the
bedside with a sheet on which the patient notes the time and amount
of drug taken. Others prefer to bring the medication to the patient at
the prescribed time.

The MG Foundation has excellent booklets which give detailed
and up to date advice on MG care. It is a good idea to keep one or two
of each of these booklets on hand in case of an emergency or hospital
stay. Many hospital units keep a file on each condition that requires
specialized nursing care. The staff appreciates up to date literature and
information that helps them to prepare care guides. If you have a local
MG support group you might make it a project to supply each nursing
unit in your local hospitals with MG care outlines.

# 9

# WHAT DO I DO NOW?

The newly diagnosed myasthenic may react with relief, shock, grief, despair, or any combination of emotions. It takes time to adjust to a chronic illness. Long cherished plans and dreams may have to be abandoned, some temporarily, others forever. For a time it may seem that the dominant focus in one's life is MG, but as adjustment comes balance can be achieved. The fact that one has MG is eventually assimilated and the necessary adaptations are made.

As the patient becomes aware of his own personal pattern, and learns to work within it, life is not so constricted. Physical limitations can usually be worked around or planned around, though many MG patients have to live with some amount of physical disability.

## GRIEF FOR "OLD" SELF

When myasthenic symptoms develop rapidly the contrast between before and after is sharp. The diagnosis may be devastating, like the sudden and unexpected death of a loved one. For a patient whose strength has gradually declined the diagnosis (at last!) may initially come as a relief, but when the sense of relief fades there is still a sense of loss.

The newly diagnosed patient may feel as if they are riding an emotional roller coaster. This is to be expected. The formerly reliable self has assumed a new and unpredictable aspect. There may be a change in roles when a wage-earner or homemaker becomes partially or totally dependent. Treatments and medications may cause pain or discomfort. It would be stressful for a healthy person to deal with. It is even more difficult to cope when in the grip of illness.

Patients often go through a grieving period similar to that associated with other kinds of loss. And, as with any loss, grief must be worked through before adjustment can be achieved.

Some patients will not allow themselves to grieve or will not acknowledge their grief. But grieving is a process, a kind of journey, which ends in adjustment. Grief follows a recognized pattern which has five stages.

## STAGE 1: DENIAL

An emotional numbness descends after any significant trauma. For a time the person may not feel anything at all, may deny that anything is wrong, or deny that what has happened has affected them deeply. This denial may be emotional, verbal or physical, as in the patient who refuses to slow down and rest, but continues to push from one crisis to another.

## STAGE 2: ANGER

"Why *me* ?" a patient may ask. "I've never been sick a day in my life!" Anger is sometimes directed at the doctor, the hospital, the medical establishment, family, friends, God, the family dog or any other nearby person or object. It's helpful to realize that this anger has its roots in frustration, disappointment, fear and emotional pain. Even when we are angry it's appropriate and necessary to let those around us know that they are not the source of our anger. Anger is something we must take personal responsibility for, and work through.

It's been taught for years that we shouldn't hold anger in, that it's better to "let it all out". But new evidence has proven that just the opposite is true. By following patients with implantable cardiac defibrillators (ICDs) cardiac researchers have learned that expressing anger is a potent trigger for heart attacks, unstable heart rhythms and strokes. Studies now show that angry outbursts put cardiac patients at risk for life-threatening events.

Since cardiac disease is the nation's number one killer most of us are potential cardiac patients. Living with unresolved anger is like living in a cage with a tiger. If you have anger issues and can't handle them on your own find an experienced counselor who can guide you.

## STAGE 3: BARGAINING

Bargaining generally doesn't last long, and may merge into the first and second stages. The futility of trying to bargain one's way out of MG is quickly apparent to most people and is soon abandoned.

## STAGE 4: DEPRESSION

Depression may arrive when we fully realize that this illness may cause long-term changes in our lives. We mourn the loss of our healthy self, and ambitions, dreams and opportunities we may have long held dear.

Depression can range from transient sadness to the total deep freeze of dysfunction. The depressed person may literally cry over spilt milk. Depression of a minor nature may not interfere with day-to-day function, but it may make life seem dull, worthless and miserable. Serious or major depression may include a number of symptoms which signal that professional help may be needed.

1. Change in sleeping patterns – sleeping far too little or too much.
2. Mood alterations which go on too long in relation to the cause.
3. Listlessness, lack of interest in things that formerly gave pleasure.
4. Inability to concentrate.
5. Eating too much or too little.
6. Inappropriate feelings of guilt.
7. Suicidal thoughts.
8. Feeling of worthlessness.
9. Loss of interest in sex or inability to have sex.
10. Lack of energy which increases over time. This can be misconstrued as "weakness" and lead to an increase in doses of Prednisone®, which can worsen the situation.

If a person has more than one or two symptoms of depression for a period of more than two weeks it is time to seek help. Prednisone® can cause mood changes, including irritability, insomnia, mania[54] and depression, and if these side effects appear they need to be addressed.

Should a person threaten or talk about suicide, or appear to be contemplating suicide, medical help should be sought immediately. The family physician may be able to give appropriate advice and guidance, but studies suggest that family physicians often overlook depression in patients. If the family physician is hesitant seek help from a mental health agency or professional.

Mild depression forces us to stretch our limits and it can be a useful prod. It may make us look for alternate solutions simply because it is such an uncomfortable and miserable state of mind. Severe depression on the other hand may cause such apathy that the

---

54 Mania: A state of extreme overactivity and high mood.

patient cannot marshal the force of will required to shake it. If depression is taking too long to resolve it may take professional help to affect the change from negative to positive, but it can be done, sometimes more quickly than thought possible. If medication proves necessary the new antidepressant medications are excellent and have far fewer side effects than older medications did.

### STAGE 5: INTEGRATION

When we have taken stock, evaluated what is left, and have determined to do the best we can with what we have, we have adjusted. Old dreams may be replaced by new ones, but these can be as much of a challenge and ultimately just as satisfying. Options may have narrowed, but while reevaluating our lives we may discover opportunities we never dreamed of before.

Every patient goes through a period of adjustment. The time it takes to adjust will vary according to the individual. Some people are resilient and bounce back quickly from the stresses of life. For others it is more of a struggle.

Joining a support group composed of other patients may help the newly diagnosed myasthenic understand and come to grips with the disease. Even if you aren't a joiner by nature it's comforting to see others coping successfully with MG. These groups also give one the opportunity to compare attitudes and coping methods, because while every individual must develop their own, it helps to see what works best for someone else.

Basically there are two ways to cope; positively or negatively. Positive methods of coping reduce anxiety, bring peace of mind and restore the patient's inner equilibrium. Negative methods cause or reinforce anxiety, isolate the patient emotionally and induce stress.

## COPING STRATEGIES

### SOME POSITIVE METHODS OF COPING INCLUDE:

#### 1. SEEKING INFORMATION

It's human nature to fear the unknown. Most patients want to know as much as possible about the disease. It's also helpful and of great emotional support to know how other patients manage. Information and peer support can be found through MG chapters, and through MG forums and chat rooms on the internet.

## 2. SPIRITUAL CONSOLATION

Gaining strength from one's spiritual values, prayer, faith communities, meditation and a belief in a benevolent Higher Power or greater purpose.

## 3. POSITIVE THINKING

Remaining optimistic, and refusing to give in to the blues. Changing one's thoughts when they become sad or fearful.

## 4. TALKING IT OUT

Verbalizing concerns, fears, anger with family, friends and other patients, seeking professional help when needed.

## 5. RECOGNIZING LIMITS

Seeking to maintain a realistic level of independence while accepting the fact that some dependence on others may be necessary.

## 6. MAINTAINING A STRONG SOCIAL NETWORK

Close ties with family, friends and a strong support network are vital to both emotional and physical health. Helping others who may have just been diagnosed or are having problems adjusting is also a healthy coping mechanism.

## 7. PHYSICAL ADAPTATION

Maximize physical capabilities by analyzing the daily routine, and adapting it to conserve energy. Learning to rest when needed, rather than push beyond your capacity.

## AMONG NEGATIVE METHODS OF COPING ARE:

## 1. DENIAL

Denial can take several forms, denying the diagnosis, non-compliance with treatment, or pushing the body too hard. There is a difference between saying, "I'm not going to let this get me down!", and "I'm not going to give in to this disease an inch!" It's healthy to do as much (or sometimes a little more) as one can. It's not healthy to consistently demand more of the body than it has to give.

## 2. BLAMING

Bitterness or anger towards oneself or someone else is not healthy. Sometimes people feel they have become ill because they were bad, or that their worth as human beings is diminished by their illness. If we look around we see that illness is part of the human condition and we are not the only one dealing with it. Moreover, anger, bitterness or guilt interfere with the process of adjustment and may weaken our ability to heal.

### 3. FOCUSING ON ILLNESS

Allowing the illness to take over and control the entire life, letting it become the main focus of the thoughts, feelings and conversation or the only factor considered in decisions.

### 4. WITHDRAWAL

Isolating oneself socially, giving up friends, interests and activities unnecessarily.

### 5. DEPRESSION

Sinking into apathy, sleeping too much or too little, engaging in obsessive behaviors, giving up on life.

### NO ONE COPES WELL ALL THE TIME

It's unrealistic to expect a person with a chronic illness to always be upbeat and optimistic, but when a person is having difficulty coping a lot of the time it is useful to look at the attitudes that characterize those who cope well and poorly.

### GENERALLY SPEAKING PEOPLE WHO COPE WELL:

1.  Are realistically optimistic about being able to cope with or solve their problems and generally maintain a high level of morale.
2.  Are practical, ready to tackle immediate problems, rather than postponing action or wishing and waiting for some magical future solution.
3.  Formulate a backup plan in case the current approach fails.
4.  Project the consequences of their actions, reasoning from cause to effect.
5.  Listen to suggestions, but retain the right to make their own decisions.
6.  Tend to be emotionally stable, avoiding emotional extremes that might impair their judgment.
7.  Are able to ask for help when they need it.

## PEOPLE WHO COPE POORLY:

1. Tend to have unrealistically high expectations for themselves and find it difficult to compromise or ask for help.
2. Tend to be intolerant; see only in black and white.
3. Tend to deny and rationalize to an excessive degree, rather than face the problem at hand.
4. Find it hard to see and weigh alternatives, and postpone making decisions until a crisis, which may worsen the situation.

These people are not necessarily ineffective in dealing with everyday life, but their inflexibility and lack of confidence hampers their ability to cope in difficult times.

## WHAT'S GOING RIGHT?

When we are under extreme stress there's a tendency to feel that everything is wrong when there are areas of life that are stable, Recognizing and drawing strength from these sources is an excellent coping mechanism.

## COPING FROM THE INSIDE OUT:

One way to cope with stress is to turn down our reaction to it. One way to do that is through meditation. Meditation has been practiced in cultures all over the world for thousands of years. It's now being used with increasing frequency by western physicians and health care organizations to treat a diverse range of medical conditions.

The purpose of meditation is to calm the mind and restore a sense of quiet. When the mind is quiet the body can restore the delicate chemical, hormonal and electrical balance that promotes health. When a person is under stress the blood pressure rises, the heart rate and respiration quicken. The immune system becomes less able to deal with invasion and more prone to self-destruction. Blood moves from the skin, hands and feet into the large muscles and vital organs.

When you're stressed your ability to think on your feet tends to vanish because the tiny capillaries in your brain clench down. Thus the blood supply to your brain, with the oxygen and nourishment it carries, is diminished during periods of stress while blood is channeled to the large muscles and heart. In many people stress is a chronic state and a significant contributor to disease states.

There are many ways to reduce stress. Exercise and vigorous physical activity are often promoted as stress reduction techniques. Unfortunately vigorous exercise is not an option for most people with MG. Even gentle exercise regimes like yoga and tai chi can be too strenuous for some MG patients.

One proven way to reduce stress which all MG patients can practice, regardless of strength level, is meditation. Over the last 25 years a whole field of investigation has grown up around the practice of meditation. It is now known that the stress response in the brain is marked by low amplitude, high frequency beta wave patterns. Meditation induces just the opposite effect in the brain, and is characterized by a state with high amplitude, low frequency alpha and theta rhythms.

Harvard University professor Herbert Benson, MD began studying meditation over 30 years ago. He soon proved that meditation can be practiced independently of any religion. The benefits of meditation are available to anyone who is willing to invest 20 minutes of daily practice. It is the practice, and not the religious intent, that brings about what Dr. Benson called the *relaxation response*. Dr. Benson has documented the uniquely altered quality of the meditative state; it's not like sleeping and not like being fully awake. Deep meditation is characterized by distinct changes in metabolism, heart rate, respiration, blood pressure and brain chemistry.

"There is significant data that meditation can enhance healing," says Saki Santorelli, director of the Center for Mindfulness in Medicine, Health Care and Society, University of Massachusetts.

So far, none of the hundreds of studies on meditation have looked specifically at MG. However, stress is associated with exacerbations in many kinds of autoimmune diseases, and many studies have shown meditation can significantly lower stress, chronic pain and anxiety.

Picture a small stream in a forest which a deer has muddied while wading across. Within a few minutes the mud, leaf litter, and debris which was stirred up by the deer has either settled, or has been swept away, leaving the stream clear. Now think of your mind as that stream. While sitting in meditation you allow your troubled thoughts, feelings and daily stress to settle or flow away, leaving your mind clear.

Meditation involves using any number of awareness techniques to quiet the mind and relax the body. Concentration practices and mindfulness meditation are perhaps the best known. These techniques focus on the silent repetition of a word, phrase, sound, or your own breathing. When attention wanders, it is gently brought back to the focus of concentration.

Meditation allows you to respond rather than simply react to situations in your daily life. Meditation can also be used to get you through unpleasant or lengthy procedures. The ability to meditate can be invaluable at such times.

Meditation is simple to learn, but not easy to practice. It takes discipline to remain still and focused, physically and mentally, for the 20 minutes of daily practice required. But this repetition and stillness are at the core of meditation and the source of its many benefits.

## HOW TO MEDITATE:

Choose a quiet spot where you will not be interrupted. If you have a timer, set it for 10 - 15 minutes.

1. Sit quietly in a comfortable position. This can be in a firm but comfortable chair, or even lying down if you are unable to sit up. But the spine should be straight. Those who need to use a chair should sit upright with their feet touching the ground with the palms of the hands resting on the thighs.
2. The eyes should not be closed but the gaze should be focused downward to rest a couple of feet in front of the nose. The gaze is soft. The object is to reduce sensory input as much as possible.
3. Take several long, deep breaths. Breathe using the diaphragm, the lower belly should fill and expand, not the chest. The breath should be relaxed, natural and quiet.
4. Relax your muscles.
5. Breathe in slowly and naturally, and begin counting silently (or aloud if you prefer). As you inhale count *one*, and as you exhale count *two* , as you inhale the next time count *three* and as you exhale count *four*. Continue counting in this manner, focusing entirely on the breath and the count until you reach 10. Then begin again, counting to 10 as you inhale and exhale. If other thoughts intrude stop counting and begin again at *one*.
6. Assume a passive attitude. Don't worry about how well you're doing. When other thoughts intrude, simply acknowledge them, and gently return to your meditation.
7. Continue for your predetermined time.
8. Sit quietly for a minute or so, allowing other thoughts to return. Focus yourself and sit for another minute before rising.

Practice this technique twice daily. Expect it to take three or four weeks before you begin to be able to keep your mind still while you count, and before you'll begin to notice significant benefits. There are many meditation techniques. You may prefer a different technique. There are many books, tapes, CDs and videos available for purchase in bookstores. Just make sure that you are buying one which is consistent with your belief system, if that is important to you. There are also meditation teachers in most towns, so if you want a personal teacher or more information, seek out local resources through community colleges or health organizations.

## LIFE ON A ROLLER COASTER

It's important to cultivate a positive self-image. Even though there may be changes in a person's capabilities to perform certain tasks, it's important to remember, "I *have* a body, but I am *not* my body." Your body may find itself strong or weak, it may be well-rested or bone-tired, but that has nothing to do with your real *self*. Your body is an instrument of experience and action, but it is only an instrument. You must treat it well, cherish it, and seek to keep it in the best of health, but never mistake it for your real self: You *have* a body, but *you* are *not* your body.

Life can sometimes be difficult for myasthenics and their families. When a family member is blind, an amputee or is disabled in a predictable way, the family knows what to expect from day-to-day. The family knows what their disabled family member can and can't do, knows what help they need, and what they can manage on their own. Unfortunately the nature of MG symptoms means that abilities vary from day to day. It's often difficult to know what help is needed. Maintaining the balance between dependence and independence is much harder than in cases where disability is consistent.

Unless they are severe, MG symptoms may not even be noticeable to the outsider. The patient may not be strong enough to stand or perform the simplest task and yet may look quite normal. Perhaps, because of the invisible nature of the disease, families tend to forget how limited the strength of the myasthenic can be. Patients (especially mothers) are frequently expected to function well beyond their physical capabilities. Many push themselves beyond their limits. Patients themselves must learn to to do what is possible independently, and ask for help when it is needed.

Though the household routine may need adaptation, every attempt should be made to maintain a sense of normal family life. The patient should be as independent as possible but they should have the necessary support in place for times when they are unable to handle daily tasks.

## You Look Wonderful!

It is sometimes disheartening for the myasthenic to hear, "But you look so well!" No one wants to look sick, but somehow it's hard not to feel defensive when it's subtly implied that you couldn't possibly be as sick as you let on. Because myasthenics do tend to look better than they feel, it's easy for others to assume that they are capable of more than they are. It takes courage, determination and creativity to lead as active and joyous a life as is possible under the circumstances. When energy is in limited supply it's wise to spend it carefully on those things that bring you and the ones you love the most happiness.

Most myasthenics can lead normal (though adapted) lifestyles. It may take time to get the disease under control, but many MG patients experience good recovery and some eventually have no symptoms at all.

It's helpful to remember that most myasthenics stabilize eventually and that many others share or have shared your battle – and have won! Attention should be focused on the positives which remain, and not on what has been put on hold or lost. The person with MG may not be able to take their children skating but can listen when they need to talk, which is more than lots of physically active people ever do. It's not what you can't do that makes you the person you are, it's what you do with what you have.

## Some Words For The Family

Having a family member with a chronic illness puts an enormous strain on family relationships. Everyone must adjust and learn to cope. Tasks not only must be reassigned and the household routine upset or interrupted, but additional time and energy may often be devoted to caring for the patient.

This may be only an inconvenience if the illness is of short duration, but when the illness is chronic the adjustments may cause serious problems. It is not unusual for marriages to break down under the additional stress of chronic illness, especially when the partner who falls ill is the woman. We have high expectations of ourselves, our partners and of marriage itself. When illness intervenes and it becomes impossible to even approach (let alone fulfill) these expectations, relationships may literally come apart.

While it may not be true for all MG patients, families often expect more of a myasthenic patient than they are able to give. Because MG is not highly visible and strength levels vary so much, it is easy to forget how disabling the illness can be. It is hard for the unaffected person to fully realize the enormous amount of effort and self-discipline it requires for the myasthenic to perform even simple daily tasks. The loss of the sense of accomplishment, and the lack of control over the illness itself, cause distress enough to most patients. Unfortunately, families often add to the psychological trauma by resenting the changes imposed by the illness.

Roles and relationships may change as the family goes through the grieving process and adapts to the reality of the situation. It is important to maintain realistic expectations, ones which allow the patient both support and independence. Some families find this a difficult process and may need to seek outside counseling. It is unrealistic to expect total patience, total self-sacrifice and unconditional acceptance of anyone. There will be good days and bad, times when the household runs smoothly and times of total chaos.

A great deal of satisfaction can be derived from working together to overcome obstacles. Difficult circumstances can bring families closer together. Unfortunately, many of us have not been taught to persevere in the face of adversity. Past generations were brought up to expect a great deal of hard work and very few comforts. They didn't anticipate easy lives. This very attitude helped them through times of hardship and crisis. Considering that life itself is full of challenges, it seems that this philosophy could be as useful to us today as it was to our ancestors.

The expression of mutual support and a determination to see the crisis through can go a long way toward cementing relationships. Family counseling can be a big help in adjusting to the changes that chronic illness brings to a home. It is very helpful if the entire family understands MG and works to minimize its impact together.

# 10

# ISSUES OF DAILY LIFE

## ASSUME RESPONSIBILITY

Access to physicians is now often limited. When you have only 10 minutes with the doctor you have to make the most of it. Organization counts! Go prepared, with a clearly written (or printed) list of your current meds, with dosages and schedule included. Make a separate list of needed refills, with the name of the medication, dose and schedule copied from a current container. Make a list of your questions and concerns in descending order, with the most urgent at the top, the second-most urgent next, etc. Address the issues in order, and if you don't get the entire list covered, at least it's the least urgent issues which get pushed to the next appointment.

## A DOCUMENTED HISTORY IS GOLD

Years ago young physicians often set up their first office on Main Street and stayed there until they retired. These days physicians migrate like hummingbirds, and there's no guarantee your medical records will be available to you (or a new physician) in five years or even six months, time. In addition more and more family physicians do not maintain hospital practices. Patients are often admitted under the care of a "Hospitalist" - a specialist who cares only for hospitalized patients.

It's important to talk to your neurologist about what to do in case of any illness which exacerbates your MG symptoms. Ask for clear *written* guidelines that tell you when to go to the emergency room, or when to call an ambulance. Patients with chronic illnesses often postpone seeking medical attention because they don't want to be a "bother" or perceived of as a complainer, but delay can prove dangerous.

When you have MG it is essential to be able to present a concise and highly accurate medical history to hospital staff. Don't count on being able to give a coherent history when you are ill, and don't rely on a relative to do it. You may not be able to talk, and your relatives may be unavailable or unable to remember details of your history and your complex medical needs.

All patients with a chronic illness need to assemble and maintain a medical file. Ask your physicians for copies of *all* test results, not just the letter reporting the opinion of the person who evaluated the test, but *a copy of the test* itself. If you have gone to the emergency department or have been admitted to the hospital, get copies of all tests done while you were there. Get copies of all your diagnostic records, including specialists' reports and letters.

Some physicians and hospitals are reluctant to give test results and reports to patients, but it is your legal right in both the USA and Canada to have a copy of your own medical records. You may be required to pay copying fees. A fee of $1.00 a page is reasonable. The $5.00 - $7.50 a page some offices and hospitals charge is too much. In such cases talk to your physician directly during a visit about your need for your records. Assure her that you are simply trying to preserve a coherent medical history. Your physician can order hospital records for you, with a signed release form.

Using your records you should prepare a document summarizing your medical history, including a list of your medications, and any allergies you have. Include your insurance information and an emergency contact. Carry two copies with you at all times. This is invaluable should you be unable to give the information to medical staff in times of crisis or emergency.

## MONITORING IS A MUST!

You must also make certain that you are followed properly when you are on the powerful medications given to MG patients. The side effects of these drugs need to be monitored periodically, even when you feel well. At one time physicians booked follow-up appointments at regular intervals. Now it may be left to the patient to make certain they see the doctor on a regular basis, and have the appropriate blood work and other tests.

It's also an excellent practice to occasionally review the official MG sites on-line. This is a good way to stay informed on any newly developing treatments, as well as gain valuable insight into MG.

## ARE YOU STILL SMOKING?

MG patients who smoke are putting themselves in a very dangerous position. Lung infections are a serious concern with myasthenics. Many myasthenic patients have breathing problems, and steroid or immune-suppression vulnerability to infection which set the stage for lung infections. Since MG patients tend to be unable to breathe deeply or cough strongly, secretions build up in the lung and form an ideal breeding ground for bacteria.

The surfaces of the bronchial tubes are covered with tiny hair-like projections called cilia. These cilia are in constant motion. They sweep accumulated bits of dust, smoke and bacteria upwards on a film of mucus, where it is all expelled from the lung by coughing. There are substances in tobacco smoke which paralyze cilia, allowing bacteria and contamination to build up in the lung, setting the stage for infection. For this reason smoking is especially hazardous for the myasthenic.

If you need to quit smoking talk to your doctor. No one need go cold turkey any more. There are a variety of aids to help smokers kick the habit, including nicotine gum, the patch, and pills to ease the craving. Most hospitals have clinics and classes to help smokers quit.

## DEALING WITH OTHER ILLNESSES

A healthy person can go to the corner drugstore and buy an over-the-counter medication to ease the discomfort of a cold, a sore back or a throbbing headache. However many over-the-counter drugs contain agents which may make myasthenic symptoms worse. Many myasthenics have ended up in crisis after taking a non-prescription hay fever pill, muscle relaxant or cough syrup. It is safest to check with your pharmacist or physician before taking any over-the-counter medication. Even then it's wise to take a very small amount the first few times to determine how much tolerance you have to the drug.

## HERBAL REMEDIES

Myasthenics need to avoid some herbal remedies, such as Siberian ginseng (aka eleuthero), aloe, burdock root, schisandra, snow fungus, cat's claw and echinacea. These herbs stimulate the immune system, and in some cases specifically stimulate the production of B cells. They make the immune attack against the NMJ stronger, when therapy in MG is directed at weakening the immune attack.

## PRESCRIPTION DRUGS

Caution is also indicated when taking prescription medication. Questions often arise as to whether certain medications should be prescribed. Patients react in individual ways to medications, depending on the combination of meds they are taking, how strong they are at the time and a host of other factors. The Myasthenia Gravis Foundation has an excellent physician's reference on drugs on their website at: http://www.myasthenia.org/drugs/reference.htm.

## D-PENICILLAMINE

One drug that should absolutely never be prescribed for a myasthenic is D-Penicillamine. This drug is used to treat rheumatoid arthritis, Wilson's disease, an inflammatory skin disorder called eosinophilic fasciitis and a few other conditions. It can cause MG in a formerly healthy person and can increase symptoms in a person with MG. (See the section on D-Pen induced myasthenia in Chapter Two.)

## AMINOGLYCOSIDE ANTIBIOTICS

The aminoglycoside antibiotics are used to treat serious bacterial infections but they are also the drugs most frequently reported to induce neuromuscular blockade in MG patients. In studies conducted on muscle sections it has been found that the aminoglycoside antibiotics substantially reduce quantal release of acetylcholine (ACh) at the axon terminal.

As well as reducing quantal release of ACh, some aminoglycosides interact post-synaptically with ion channels on the AChR in their open configuration. Others block AChR receptors. These actions provide an explanation for the neuromuscular block these antibiotics produce and the resulting weakness observed in the MG patient. Neomycin has the most potent neuromuscular blocking action of these drugs.

## GENERIC AND BRAND NAMES OF AMINOGLYCOSIDE ANTIBIOTICS: (TABLE 10:1)

| Table 10.1 | |
|---|---|
| **Aminoglycoside Generic Name** | **Aminoglycoside Brand Name(s)** |
| Amikacin | Amikin® |

| Table 10.1 | |
|---|---|
| **Aminoglycoside Generic Name** | **Aminoglycoside Brand Name(s)** |
| Gentamicin | Garamycin® |
| Kanamycin | Kantrex® |
| Neomycin | Mycifradin®, NeoTab® Myciguent®, |
| Netilmicin | Netromycin® |
| Paromomycin | Humatin® |
| Tobramycin | AKTob®,Tobrex®,Nebcin®, Tobradex®,TOBI Solution® |
| Streptomycin sulfate, Streptomycin nitrate | Streptomycin® |

## OTHER ANTIBIOTICS (TABLE 10:2)

Other antibiotics which have caused problems in some MG patients include those in the following table. The majority of MG patients can take these antibiotics without any problems.

| Table 10.2 | |
|---|---|
| **Antibiotic Generic Name** | **Antibiotic Brand Name(s)** |
| Azithromycin | Zithromax® |
| Ciprofloxacin | Ciloxan®, Cipro® |
| Clindamycin | Cleocin® |
| Colistin | Cortisporin-TC Otic Suspension[55] ® |
| Erythromycin | E-Mycin®, Eryc®, Ery-Tab®, PCE®, Pediazole®, Ilosone® |
| Lincomycin | Lincocin®, Lincorex® |

---

55 Cortisporin – TC Otic Suspension: Colistin, neomycin and corticosteroid mixture which is used in the ear to treat bacterial infections.

| Table 10.2 | |
|---|---|
| **Antibiotic Generic Name** | **Antibiotic Brand Name(s)** |
| Metronidazole | Flagyl® |
| Metronidazole/Nystatin | Flagystatin® |
| Polymyxin B | Polymyxin B® |
| Tetracycline | Achromycin®, Actisite®, Sumycin®, Topicycline® |

### INTERFERON ALPHA

Interferon alpha is a man-made copy of antigens made naturally by the immune system. The body makes interferon as part of its response to infection or cancer. Interferon is used to treat several types of cancer, particularly renal cell (kidney cancer), malignant melanoma, multiple myeloma and some types of leukemia. It is also used to treat diseases other than cancer; diabetes, Karposi's sarcoma in AIDs, growths in the respiratory tract in children called laryngeal papillomatosis, and some kinds of hepatitis.

AChR antibody positive MG has developed in some people who received interferon alpha treatment. Some MG patients also had worsening of MG symptoms after interferon alpha treatment. Other reports document the successful treatment of cancer in MG patients with low-dose interferon alpha, with no exacerabation of MG symptoms. In these cases all the available medical information has to be reviewed very carefully by patient, neurologist and others on the medical team. Brand names of Interferon include: Alferon N®, Roferon-A®, Intron A®, and in Canada, an additional brand name, Wellferon®.

### MUSCLE RELAXANTS, TRANQUILIZERS AND ANTIDEPRESSANTS

#### LITHIUM:

There are reports that MG developed in some patients who were being treated with lithium. Some cases seemed to be the result of the lithium itself, one appeared to be a mild case of MG which was exacerbated by the lithium.

## MUSCLE RELAXANTS

Muscle relaxants and tranquilizers can have an exaggerated effect on a myasthenic and should be taken with caution. Some authorities recommend initially using a tenth of the normal dose of muscle relaxants and tranquilizers in MG patients.

## ANTIDEPRESSANTS

Some MG patients also report increased weakness when using the tricyclic antidepressants Elavil®, Sinequan® or Tofranil®. Although there are no reports in medical literature on the effects of the serotonin reuptake inhibitors (SSRI) anti-depressants Prozac®, Paxil® and Celexa® on MG patients, studies show that fluoxetine (Prozac®) both blocks AChRs and increases the rate at which which they desensitize.

## BETA BLOCKERS, SODIUM CHANNEL BLOCKERS, CALCIUM CHANNEL BLOCKERS AND ANTI-ARRHYTHMICS

MG patients are as likely as anyone to develop other health problems. MG patients and their physicians are often faced with the need to choose medication to treat high blood pressure or a heart condition.

High blood pressure and erratic or irregular heart rhythms are usually treated with drugs which block various ion channels in cell membranes – hence their names; beta blockers, calcium channel blockers and sodium channel blockers. Blocking specific ion channels can lower (or raise) blood pressure, and alter the rhythm and force of the heartbeat. A side effect of many of these drugs is that they can also cause weakness of skeletal muscle.

## BETA BLOCKERS

Beta adrenergic receptors are part of the body's communication system. These receptors respond to epinephrine, a hormone secreted by the adrenal gland. When epinephrine binds to sites on the beta receptors the heart rate and the force of the heartbeat increase, blood pressure increases and bronchial muscles relax. In other words, the body gets ready to react quickly to stress.

Beta blockers bind to beta-1 receptor sites, which control circulation primarily in the heart. This lowers the stimulation level by lowering the number of potential binding sites for epinephrine. Beta blockers don't cause serious deterioration for most MG patients, but they are reported to cause increased fatigue and occasional double vision, even in patients without MG. They have been reported with worsening symptoms in some MG patients, though one experienced clinician says he has never seen a case where propranolol worsened MG symptoms.

## GENERIC AND BRAND NAMES OF BETA BLOCKERS: (TABLE 10:3)

| Table 10.3 Beta Blockers Generic Name | Beta Blockers Brand Names |
|---|---|
| Atenolol | Atenolol®, Tenormin®, Atenolol/CHLO®, Tenoretic 50®, Tenoretic 100® |
| Labetalol | Normodyne®, Trandate® |
| Metoprolol | Lopressor®, Toprol XL® |
| Nadolol | Corgard® |
| Oxprenolol | Oxprenolol Hydrochloride®, Coretal®, Koretal®, Trasicor®, Slow Trasicor®, Tevacor® |
| Practolol | Eralzdin Practolol®, Dalzic® |
| Propranolol | Inderal®, Inderal-LA®, Inderide®, Inderide-LA®, Propranolol-HCL® |
| Timolol | Timolide®, Blocadren® |

## SODIUM CHANNEL BLOCKERS

Quinidine and procainamide regulate the flow of sodium ions into heart cells. Sodium channel blockers slow the inward rush of sodium ions and make the heart less vulnerable to erratic rhythms, but quinidine has such an effect on AChRs, and on alpha binding sites in particular, that it is used as a therapy in Slow Channel Myasthenic Syndrome. In Slow Channel Syndrome the sodium ion channels remain open too long, resulting in muscle weakness and damage that accumulates over time. Quinidine makes patients with Slow Channel Syndrome better because it closes the ion channels more quickly. In a healthy person this doesn't pose a problem, but in the person with autoimmune MG it poses a significant risk. In fact, quinidine's post-synaptic effects are described as *curare-like*, which is to say they can cause paralysis.

Procainamide has similar effects. There is a case in medical literature of an MG patient with no prior history of respiratory weakness who experienced respiratory failure requiring intubation immediately after receiving procainamide. When the drug wore off, the patient's strength returned, and he was able to breathe on his own again.

Typical doses of procainamide decrease miniature endplate potentials (MEPPs) without altering resting membrane potential. However, the typical dose causes a reduction in the number of quanta of ACh released at the axon terminal, a reduction in the amplitude of impulse-evoked end-plate potentials (EPPs) and a marked prolongation of the decaying phase. This translates into less stimulation for AChRs. This can be dangerous for MG patients.

## SODIUM CHANNEL BLOCKERS GENERIC AND BRAND NAMES (TABLE 10:4)

| Table 10.4 Sodium Channel Blockers Generic Names | Sodium Channel Blockers Brand Names |
|---|---|
| Procainamide | Pronestyl®, Procan-SR®, Procanbid®, Procan SR®, Pronestyl-SR® |
| Quinidine | Quinaglute®, Quinaglute-Dura-tabs®, Quinidex®, Quinidex Extentabs®, Quinora®, Cardioquin®, Quin-Release® <br><br> In Canada— Apo-Quinidine® Biquin Durules®, Quinate®, Novoquinidin® |

Quinidine and quinine are related and can be dangerous to the person with MG, so one would naturally expect to avoid these drugs. But *tonic water*, a popular mixer for alcoholic beverages, is on every grocer's shelf. Tonic water may contain enough quinine to cause significant weakness in some patients.

## CALCIUM CHANNEL BLOCKERS

Calcium channel blockers slow the flow of calcium ions into the heart muscle and blood vessel walls. This relaxes the blood vessels so that blood flows more easily through them, and less pumping force is required from the heart, thereby lowering blood pressure. For this reason calcium channel blockers are used to treat high blood pressure, angina[56], and cardiac arrhythmia[57]. Calcium channel blockers affect neuromuscular transmission in ways which may make MG and LEMS patients weaker.

Verapamil is a calcium channel blocker which has effects on both pre-synaptic and post-synaptic voltage-dependent calcium channels at the NMJ. In an MG or LEMS patient who has just had surgery oral verapamil can cause a marked worsening of myasthenic symptoms. Verapamil has also caused respiratory failure in an MG patient.

In one surgical study verapamil was administered to five MG patients, and 12 patients without neuromuscular diseases, while they were anesthetized, and the effect on muscle strength was observed. Verapamil produced significant neuromuscular blocking action in the MG patients. The researchers concluded that caution is needed when administering verapamil to MG patients.

Not all neurologists believe that verapamil worsens symptoms in MG, and feel that experience has shown verapamil is an acceptable drug in MG.

## CALCIUM CHANNEL BLOCKER GENERIC AND BRAND NAMES: (TABLE 10.5)

| Table 10.5 Calcium Channel Blockers Generic Name | Calcium Channel Blockers Brand Names |
|---|---|
| Amlodipine | Lotrel®, Norvasc® |

---

56 Angina: Heart muscle pain that comes with exertion.
57 Cardiac arrhythmia: Erratic or irregular heart rhythms.

| Table 10.5 Calcium Channel Blockers Generic Name | Calcium Channel Blockers Brand Names |
|---|---|
| Bepridil | Vascor® |
| Diltiazem | Cardizem®,Cardizem-CD®, Cardizem-SR®,Dilacor-XR®, Cartia®, Diltia-XT® ,Tiamate®, Tiazac® (Canada)Apo-Diltiaz,® Cardizem®,Cardizem-SR®, Novo-Diltazem®,Nu-Diltiaz®, Syn-Diltiazem®, |
| Felodipine | Plendil® (Canada) Renedil® |
| Flunarizine | (Canada) Sibelium® |
| Isradipine | DynaCirc® |
| Nicardipine | Cardene® |
| Nifedipine | Adalat®, Procardia-XL®, Procardia®, In Canada – Apo-Nifed®,Novo-Nifedin®, NuNifed® |
| Nimodipine | Nimotop® |
| Nisoldipine | Sular® |
| Nitrendipine | Cardif®, Nitrepin® |
| Verapamil | Calan®, Covera-HS®, Isoptin®, Verelan® (Canada) Apo-Verap®, Novo-Veramil®, Nu-Verap® |
| Combination of Verapamil and Trandolapril | Tarka® |

## LOCAL ANESTHETICS

The occasional MG patient reacts badly to Novocaine® (xylocaine), a local anesthetic used for dental work or minor surgeries. Novocaine® is chemically related to procainamide. If you have had weakness associated with Novocaine® ask for a local anesthetic which is unrelated to procainamide.

## DIURETICS

Diuretics are used to treat high blood pressure and congestive heart failure because they cause excretion of excess fluid. Diuretics like Lasix® and Hydrodiuril® may cause muscle cramps and increase weakness in MG patients, possibly because they cause increased excretion of potassium. Some diuretics cause the kidneys to hold onto potassium, (Aldactone®, Spironolactone®). MG patients who need a diuretic might discuss using one of these with their physician.

## ANALGESICS , ANTICONVULSANTS AND BARBITURATES

Analgesics like morphine and Leritine® should be used with caution in MG patients with breathing or swallowing problems because they cause suppression of the breathing reflex. There have been reports of patients who developed MG while taking the anti-convulsant drugs Dilantin® (phenytoin), Mesantoin® (mephenytoin) or Tridione® (trimethadione). Some of these cases of MG disappeared when the drugs were discontinued. It is possible that these patients already had mild MG which was made worse by the medications, and which subsided without the medication.

Dilantin® increases the spontaneous release of individual molecules of ACh at the axon terminal (increasing MEPPs), while reducing quantal release of ACh (reducing EPPs). Reducing EPPs lowers the force of muscle contraction.

Gabapentin (Neurotin®), prescribed for seizures and nerve pain, has been reported to both precipitate and exacerbate autoimmune MG when prescribed for as short a period as three months. After MG was observed in patients treated with gabapentin, a study was conducted in rats with MG. When a *single* dose of gabapentin was given to rats with experimentally induced MG it caused temporary muscle weakness within three hours. It is recommended by the authors of these reports that gabapentin should be used with caution in MG.

## BARBITURATES

There's only a single report in the literature of barbiturates exacerbating MG weakness, but numerous patients of this author's acquaintance have reported weakness associated with barbiturate drugs. Barbiturates are central nervous system (CNS) depressants. Some barbiturates are used before surgery to relieve anxiety or tension. Some are used to help control seizures. Barbiturates are sometimes included as ingredients of other drugs, such as in the commonly prescribed pain relievers Fiorinal® (a combination of aspirin, barbiturate and caffeine) and Fioricet® (acetaminophen, barbiturate and caffeine).

### COMMON BRAND AND GENERIC NAMES OF BARBITURATES: (TABLE 10:6)

| Table 10.6 Barbiturates Generic Name | Barbiturates Brand Names |
|---|---|
| Amobarbital | Amytal® |
| Aprobarbital | Alurate® |
| Butabarbital | Busodium®, Butalan®, Butisol®, Sarisol No. 2® |
| Butabital + aspirin +caffeine | Fiorinal® |
| Butabital+acetaminophen +caffeine | Fioricet® |
| Mephobarbital | Mebaral® |
| Pentobarbital (Canada) | Nembutal®, Novopentobarb®, Nova Rectal® |
| Phenobarbital | Barbital®, Luminal®, Solfoton®, Nembutal®, (Canada) Ancalixir® |
| Secobarbital | Seconal® (Canada) Novosecobarb® |
| Secobarbital & Amobarbital | Tuinal® |

## MEDICATIONS AND SAFETY

The best strategy for managing medications is for the MG patient to work with their neurologist, but there are many times when the family physician, or another caregiver, prescribes medications for other health conditions. If at all possible it's best to coordinate care between caregivers, but there are times when this is impossible. If asked, the neurologist may be willing to recommend a list of antibiotics, or other medications for which the need might arise, that the patient can carry along with their medical information.

### CHECKING FOR SIDE EFFECTS OF PRESCRIPTION DRUGS

You have every right to ask that any drug you are prescribed be checked in the *CPS (Compendium of Pharmaceuticals and Specialties)* in Canada or the *PDR (Physician's Desk Reference)* in the U.S.A. These are references all physicians and pharmacists have. Your doctor should be willing to do this for you, but your pharmacist should also be willing to look up medication for you *before* the prescription is filled. The CPS is at hand in every pharmacy. Most pharmacists will allow you to read the section pertaining to the drug in question. If you don't understand the technical language ask for an explanation.

You can also look the drug up on the Internet. You can use a search engine to look up the drug's generic or brand name. Simply type the name in the search box. Or you can go to one of the sites below and look the drug's name up there. If you are looking for a good basic explanation in layman's language go to the National Institutes of Health Medline Plus Drug Information site:

http://www.nlm.nih.gov/medlineplus/druginformation.html.

If you want more detailed information try http://www.rxlist.com.

When researching a drug for use by a myasthenic, look for certain terms. In the *Contraindications*[58] section look for the phrases "contraindicated for patients with myasthenia gravis" or the phrase "patients with active neurological disorders" or "patients with a history of respiratory depression or respiratory failure[59]".

---

58 Contraindications: Don't give this drug to patients with the conditions listed in this section.

59 Respiratory depression or failure: An inability to breathe adequately without assistence.

There may be a section under *Adverse Effects* that says CNS (central nervous system). Look for weakness, fatigue, respiratory depression or disturbances. If you can't remember all the terms, write them on a card and slip them in your wallet.

Pharmacists are expected to know the side effects of all prescription drugs. Your pharmacist should be aware that you have MG, and that your condition makes you sensitive to the effects of neuromuscular blocks and CNS depressants. If there is a question about the potential effect on a drug on your strength level or respiratory capacity, it is acceptable (even desirable), for the pharmacist to call the physician with the concern.

When checking out medications yourself **it is important to remember** that information on the web or even in the CPS is not always up-to-date. Some drugs once believed to be dangerous to myasthenics are now considered safe because of wider experience and knowledge. It's always best to discuss new medications with your neurologist whenever possible.

## MEDIC ALERT AND "ICE"

The MG patient should wear a medical alert bracelet or necklace and carry a one-page medical history. This history should contain a drug caution warning that the use of muscle relaxants, neuromuscular blocks (including curare and curare-like muscle relaxants), Quinidine®, Procainamide® and other antiarrhythmics can cause CNS or respiratory depression.

If you have a cell phone you can program in an emergency contact person's number under the acronym *ICE* for "In Case of Emergency". This way if you cannot speak for yourself in an emergency paramedics immediately have a contact number available.

## NORMALIZING EVERYDAY LIFE

Heat is weakening for some myasthenics, while others report that cold weakens them. Symptoms may be much worse during very hot or cold weather. It's best, if possible, to avoid extremes of temperature. If heat is weakening cool showers are better than hot baths. In fact, many myasthenics report that the response of facial muscles can be improved if the face is washed with cold water. Cold or cool food and drink are often easier to chew and swallow than the same items heated.

## PACE NOT RACE

Common sense suggests that patients learn to pace themselves, alternating activity with sedentary pursuits or rest periods. The price of doing more than you should physically is high, and it may take several days to recover. Squandering strength on relatively unimportant tasks or activities only means that there will be less left to spend on those activities that are truly important.

## CLOTHING

Clothing can be selected for ease of care and for ease when dressing. Coats, shoes and boots should be lightweight and practical. Shoes should support the foot and have low, stable heels. Zippered or Velcro® closings make shoes easier to get on and off. Elastic shoelaces can make it possible to slide laced shoes off and on. A long-handled shoehorn is a help. Buttons can be done up with an old-fashioned button-hook. It's less tiring to dress if clothing can be pulled or slipped on. Allow extra time when dressing, because you may need a short rest after. It's been said in jest, but with ring of truth, that the myasthenic can get ready to go - or go - but not both!

## AIDS FOR INDEPENDENCE

Satin or silky pajamas and satin sheets reduce resistance and make it easier to turn over or move easily in bed. Raising the bed a few inches can make getting in and out of bed easier, and can also ease making the bed, because you don't have to bend over as far.

In the bathroom, a clip-on raised toilet seat can be helpful if the patient has difficulty rising from a seated position. Supports can be placed on either side of the toilet, or a grab bar can be attached to the vanity, if it is nearby and sturdy enough. If grooming is done at the bathroom vanity, a barstool or stool-height chair may make it easier. A dressing table and chair are an alternate choice. Grooming supplies should be kept at the lowest level feasible, so that there is no need to reach up. A mirror which sits on the counter surface, so the person can look down, rather than up, is much less fatiguing.

The bathtub should have a nonskid bottom and firmly attached grab bars to prevent falls. A shower chair is helpful if the patient has trouble standing or getting out of the tub. There should be a non-skid bathmat on the floor.

There's a toothbrush specially designed for people who have strength issues or are otherwise disabled. It's called the Collis Curve®. This brush has two outer rows of soft bristles curved around a center row of short, stiff ones. This design minimizes position changes needed for effective brushing and improves ease of access to harder-to-reach teeth. The Collis brush has been shown to reduce plaque in half the time required with conventional toothbrushes, which makes it easier to use for those whose arms fatigue quickly. Our Collis brushes came from our dentist, but Collis-Curve® brushes can be ordered directly from the company. (See the Appendix)

## GET A GRIP!

It takes more force to maintain a grip on a small-diameter object than on a large-diameter one, so it can be helpful to increase the diameter of items like toothbrushes and hairbrushes. Specialized grips can be purchased at medical supply stores. Home supply stores carry a type of inexpensive dense tubular foam that is used to insulate water pipes. This inexpensive foam is just as effective as the expensive grips. This tubing has an inner diameter of either ½" or ¾" . It has a split down one side so it can be opened and slipped over small-sized handles. It can also be used to increase the diameter of spoons, forks and kitchen utensils. If doorknobs pose a problem they can be replaced by lever type handles.

## KITCHEN AIDS AND CLEANERS

There are many aids which can make household, and especially kitchen chores, easier. A microwave oven drastically cuts meal preparation time and reduces the number of pans and dishes to be washed. Next on the list of must-haves are an electric can opener and a food processor. Heavy pans can be replaced by lightweight (non-stick) ones. Pans and other often-used utensils can be placed on a butcher's cart. A cart or trolley can be used to transport dishes and food from the kitchen to the table. Cooking ingredients can be bought, stored or repackaged in small containers.

Some MG patients report that exposure to household cleaning products worsens weakness. Most often mentioned are aerosol products or heavily perfumed cleaning products. Other reported precipitants of weakness are perfume and perfumed products like scented candles and soaps, potpourris and room deodorizers.

## DELEGATE!

Housekeeping standards may need to be relaxed from pre-myasthenia days. Children can be a big help with housekeeping. Mom shouldn't feel guilty about asking family members to help keep the household running smoothly. In the business world the ability to delegate is considered the sign of a good manager.

Children need to learn how to cook and keep house, so they will be able to care for themselves and their own homes in the future. Be appreciative of your family's efforts to help, and make certain they understand that the work they do is really important to you.

Family members should always be thanked for their efforts to keep the home running smoothly, even when the results aren't perfect. Praise and reward every effort, and remember, that in 25 years you want their memories to be happy ones of working together, not of screaming fights over whether the socks were folded *exactly* the way Mom liked them folded.

## OUT AND ABOUT

Some MG patients who drive may be eligible for a permit which allows use of parking spaces designated for the handicapped. Applications for handicapped parking permits usually must be signed by your physician.

## ON THE JOB

When the myasthenic works outside the home conserving energy and getting enough rest during the workday is vital. It may be possible to manage three half-hour rest periods during the day by reducing an hour-long lunch break to half an hour, then adding 15 minutes to each 15 minute coffee break. It might be easier to eat lunch at your work station or in a nearby lunchroom rather than go out somewhere which would require a long walk.

For many MG patients working outside the home is only a dream. Some are able to find work they can do at home, thus conserving the energy and strength spent on commuting, and using it for work. This is much more possible than it was 10 years ago due to the advent of the Internet and the computerization of business. In some areas there are government or agency-sponsored programs that aid disabled people in exploring employment options. Contact your local employment office to see if such programs exist in your area.

## THERE'S NO NEED TO BE ALONE

When a principal wage-earner must give up their job due to illness it can be a doubly difficult time. Not only must the patient deal with illness but with the psychological trauma that the loss of job and earning power entails. This may mean financial hardship for the family, a change of homes, schools and friends. It's a time when every emotional resource a family has can be stretched to the limit. These times can tear a family apart or knit one together so strongly that nothing can shake it. Don't face your storm alone. There are others facing the same issues and there's strength in numbers. Reach out . You don't need to be alone. Several organizations offer resources to MG patients. They are listed below.

## ORGANIZATIONS OF INTEREST TO MYASTHENICS

**Canada:**
Muscular Dystrophy Canada
2345 Yonge Street Suite 901
Toronto, Ontario M4P 2E5
Phone: 1-800 567-2873 ext.160
Website: http://muscle.ca/

Myasthenia Gravis Ontario Chapter
1317 Hixon Street, Oakville, Ontario L6L 1R5
Telephone: (905) 827-1957
Email: mgontchptr@cogeco.ca

The MG Wellness Resource Network
Iris Biteen - Phone: (514) 398-5358
e-mail: mgresource@hotmail.com

MG Manitoba Inc.
Verna Kapkey, Founder and past president
204-586-6784
e-mail: vkapkey@mts.net

Myasthenia Gravis Association of British Columbia
2805 Kings Way
Vancouver, British Columbia,
V5R 5H9
(604) 451-5511 FAX (604) 451-5651

**THE USA:**

Myasthenia Gravis Foundation of America
1821 University Ave. W., Suite S256
St. Paul, MN 55104
Telephone - (651) 917-6256 or (800) 541-5454
Web site: http://www.myasthenia.org/
Listing of all MGFA Chapters:
http://www.myasthenia.org/chapters/mgfchap1.htm

The Muscular Dystrophy Association USA
3300 East Sunrise Drive, Tucson, AZ, 85718
(602) 572-1717
Web site: http://www.mdausa.org

Myasthenia Gravis Foundation of California
5675 Telegraph Road, Suite 230
Los Angeles, California 90040
(800) 574-7884 (Toll free for California and Nevada)
Email: mgfcc@concentric.net

**INTERNET RESOURCES:**

MGnet; The Internet Chapter of the Myasthenia Gravis Foundation
http://mgfa-mgnet.org/

Bette Swann's Club of Hearts – Listserv and nightly chats
http://health.groups.yahoo.com/group/bettesmyastheniagravissupport/
Known as the Club of Hearts for its kind and caring community.

Maddy's MG Support
http://health.groups.yahoo.com/group/maddysmgsupport/
A place for people with MG to find support, encouragement, and
caring friends.

Congenital Myasthenia On-line Support Group
http://health.groups.yahoo.com/group/congenitalmyastheniagravis/
A place for those who wish to discuss CMG and related issues.

# 11

# MG – A Difficult Diagnosis

Myasthenia gravis is sometimes a difficult diagnosis to pin down. All too often, MG patients are first diagnosed as having a psychiatric illness such as conversion disorder or somatic disorder. Receiving a psychiatric diagnosis leads to significant delays in obtaining a proper diagnosis and effective treatment. Misdiagnosis continues to be a problem with MG. A recent journal article states, "In as many as 25 - 50% of patients diagnosed [with] conversion [disorder], an organic medical diagnosis was found."[60]

## The Psychiatric Misdiagnosis

A study of 200 MG patients revealed that 20% of them initially received a psychiatric misdiagnosis, with young women at higher risk of psychiatric misdiagnosis, and men more often receiving a "somatic" misdiagnosis. Somatization is the conversion of psychic pain into physical symptoms. Somatization disorder has very well-defined diagnostic criteria (see Appendix). *All* of the diagnostic criteria must be met before the diagnosis of somatization can be made. Too often the diagnosis of somatization is made based on muscle weakness *alone*.

This study points out that patients who are misdiagnosed have higher depression scores, which isn't particularly surprising. A patient with MG seeks help only to be told that their weakness is psychiatric in origin. They are then given antidepressants which increase their muscle weakness. Some patients in this situation have been told that their increased weakness indicates that they are "fighting the therapy". Many people would become depressed in such a situation.

---

60 Spinal Cord. 2002 Jul;40(7):327-34. See References, Chapter 11.

In one survey of MG patients a third of them had initially been given a psychiatric diagnosis because their symptoms fluctuated so much that there were often no abnormalities on examination, especially if the exam was conducted in the morning.

MG patients who receive a diagnosis of psychiatric illness are often resentful once their MG is diagnosed. While most realize that stress can worsen MG symptoms, almost all are upset when it is implied that this indicates that they have psychiatric problems.

## A CHICKEN AND EGG QUESTION

Some studies have suggested that MG patients are more likely than unaffected people to suppress anger and anxiety. Researchers interviewed MG patients with cases of from three months to three years duration. They concluded that persons who suppress anger and anxiety are more likely to develop MG. It apparently never occurred to them that MG patients deliberately avoid emotional outbursts after learning that these can dramatically worsen symptoms.

Thankfully, as medical science learns more, this theory is becoming less popular, but some physicians seem intent on labeling all patients with muscle weakness as psychiatric patients. Patients sometimes complain that they can't win. Their dilemma could be summed up by the words of one patient, diagnosed by the second neurologist she was sent to.

> "I went to the neurologist for the first time, and in the course of the interview, while trying to explain the detrimental effect my weakness was having on my marriage and career, I began to cry.
>
> The neurologist reported to my family doctor that he felt my weakness was emotional in origin, possibly a hysterical reaction to conflicts at home.
>
> On a second visit to this same neurologist I made sure that I remained very calm as I described my symptoms. I did not cry, and I answered his questions without elaborating on them. The report came back that my weakness was probably emotional in origin, as I was certainly not concerned about it. After that my family doctor referred me to a different neurologist, who did several tests, finding that I was anti-AChR antibody positive, and I was diagnosed."

# 12

# CASE STUDIES AND PATIENTS' COMMENTS

When I was writing the first edition of this book I included a series of comments from a group of individual patients, feeling that they might be helpful to other patients. This part of the book received a highly positive response, as other patients felt a sense of relief in knowing that they weren't alone in their day-to-day struggles.

In this edition I am adding case histories from several patients. Some summarized their experiences through a questionnaire, others wrote their experiences in more detail. I am grateful to these individuals, who have generously shared their stories with us. They give us a human perspective not found in journal articles and textbook summaries.

## AUTOIMMUNE MG - GENERALIZED SYMPTOMS

## PATIENT "A"

"A" began having symptoms of MG at age 43. When she responded to these questions she was 49 years old. She has anti-AChR antibody positive MG with ocular and generalized symptoms. Her first symptoms were a drooping left eyelid, weak neck, shoulder and arm muscles. She also experienced choking. From the time she sought medical help until she received diagnosis was two months. She saw four physicians during the diagnostic process. Tests used in the diagnostic process included EMG, Repetitive Nerve Stimulation, anti-AChR antibody, chest X-ray. and a CAT scan.

SYMPTOMS: "A" has experienced the following symptoms: droopy lids, inability to open eyes, double vision, wandering or bouncing eye, weak, crooked or flat smile, nasal and weak speech, choking, difficulties chewing and swallowing, weak neck muscles, an inability to support her head, weak hand, shoulder and arm muscles, which made tasks using those muscles difficult, foot drop, generalized fatigue, mental lethargy, pain and depression.

**TREATMENTS:** "A" has received the following treatments since diagnosis; Mestinon®, Prednisone®, Imuran®, plasmapherisis, and thymectomy. She also had the amalgam (mercury) fillings removed from her teeth. Currently she takes Mestinon® as needed, plus Prednisone® and Imuran®.

**CURRENT LEVEL OF SYMPTOMS:** In the past 12 months she has experienced severe (generalized profound) weakness for one to three days a month. She has moderate weakness which leaves her unable to carry on with daily activities one to three days a week. She has mild weakness which allows her to carry on with her activities with some difficulty three to six days a week. She has very mild weakness which doesn't interfere with activity one to three days a week. She says that treatment and management strategies have reduced the frequency and severity of her symptoms by 50 - 75%.

**AVAILABILITY OF MG INFORMATION:** Her physicians provided her with some information about MG. She was made aware that she could obtain information through the National MG Foundation. She was included in discussions about her treatment and feels that the medical care she received was mostly supportive.

## PATIENT "L":

"L" is a male patient, who developed MG symptoms at age 38, and is now 80 years old. He was diagnosed by EMG, repetitive nerve stimulation, single fiber EMG, a Tensilon® test and a positive anti-AChR antibody test. His first symptoms were facial weakness, ptosis, neck weakness and difficulties with chewing. It took two or three months from the time he sought medical help until he received his diagnosis. He saw only one physician during the diagnostic process.

**SYMPTOMS:** "L's" symptoms have included droopy lids, double vision, a weak smile, speech problems, chewing and swallowing difficulties, weak neck muscles, an inability to support his head, weak shoulder muscles which made it difficult to hold his arms above his head and weakness in his arms and hands which made it hard to maintain a grip or sustain activity. He has been unable to climb stairs at times, and has experienced generalized fatigue.

**TREATMENTS:** "L" has received the following treatments over the years: Mestinon®, prednisone, Imuran®, plasmapherisis and thymectomy. Currently he takes 60 mg. of Mestinon® three times a day and 25 mg. of Prednisone® every other day.

**CURRENT LEVEL OF SYMPTOMS:** "L" now has very mild weakness which does not interfere with his daily routine. Treatment has reduced the severity of his symptoms by 75 - 100%.

**AVAILABILITY OF MG INFORMATION:** "L's" physicians gave him the information he needed during the diagnostic and treatment process. He was told how to contact the MG Foundation. He was included in discussions about his treatment and his medical care was supportive.

## PATIENT "M'S" STORY

"In February 1973, when I was 20 years old, I began seeing double. I sought out an ophthalmologist who immediately suspected myasthenia. He arranged for me to see a neurologist who specialized in MG. After undergoing a series of tests, I responded positively to the Tensilon® test and within two weeks my diagnosis was confirmed. The doctor prescribed Mestinon® to relieve my double vision but I was not made aware that myasthenia might affect other muscles.

At the end of April I began to have difficulty chewing and climbing stairs. On the day after my 21st birthday, I was admitted to the hospital to undergo a thymectomy. My condition rapidly deteriorated, but it was two weeks before I could have the operation. As I waited my weakness progressed. I was terrified. At that time, neither plasmapherisis nor IVIG were available. Undergoing the surgery in this weakened state placed me at increased risk.

After the surgery, my condition deteriorated. I was affected in *all* muscles: eyes, eyelids, chewing, swallowing, tongue, upper palate, neck, chest, arms, hands and legs. We waited with anticipation, hoping for some sign of recovery resulting from the thymectomy. I subsisted on alternate doses of Mestinon® and Prostigmine®.

Six weeks passed with no improvement. My neurologist returned from holiday to find me still hospitalized, virtually paralyzed and immobile. Fearing that my muscles might soon atrophy, he began a more aggressive treatment, a small dose of Prednisone®, every second day, gradually increasing the dosage. It was impossible to know that the Prednisone® was masking an infection. One cool summer day, my lung collapsed without warning. I had contracted pneumonia. For the next two weeks it was touch-and-go in intensive care. It was a hellish experience – one that I will never forget. For me, MG is a life-threatening disease.

My mother had a sister who also had MG. She was diagnosed at the age of 13 and died when she was 24 years old. When my mother first heard of my diagnosis, she decided to withhold this information to protect me. How fortunate that she did. I don't think I would have survived with this knowledge.

I remained in the hospital for four months and when I returned to "normal" life pumped full of cortisone, I no longer knew who I was or what my life would be. My doctor's parting words were, "Normal people have a dollar's worth of energy each day, you will have just 50 cents." I was barely 21 years old with my whole life ahead of me! Infuriated by this life sentence, I determined to find a way to beat the odds. After an extensive five year search, I encountered Nichiren Buddhism. I knew at once that I had found the means to establish a full and active life.

It would be impossible for me to speak of my experience with MG without mentioning my Buddhist practice – the two are intertwined. In Nichiren Buddhism we chant Nam Myoho Renge Kyo. It is the source of unlimited life force and chanting enables us to tap this life force. Struggling with the fatigue of the disease compounded by the exhaustion caused by immunosuppressant drugs, I actively used the "tool" of chanting Nam Myoho Renge Kyo to strengthen my life and on many occasions, to "make the impossible possible".

After nearly six years on Prednisone®, I developed cataracts which necessitated a switch to Imuran®. In 1979, it was believed to be dangerous to administer Prednisone® and Imuran® simultaneously. As I withdrew from Prednisone® my MG symptoms resurfaced. My doctor cautioned me that because Imuran® is slow acting, we might also need to consider plasmapherisis. I chanted vigorously for the medication to take effect. Within six weeks my MG symptoms began to diminish and I achieved a full remission.

I began to experience severe side effects from the Imuran®. An exhaustive search for relief led me to an exceptionally gifted chiropractor. After ten chiropractic treatments I slowly withdrew from Imuran® and for the first time since the onset of the illness, I enjoyed a medication-free remission, which I maintained for 14 months.

That autumn I caught the flu and six weeks later, to my great disappointment, I was once again experiencing ocular symptoms. Initially I managed with Mestinon®, but within eight months the weakness spread to my arms and legs. Recalling the painful side effects of Imuran®, I still put off further treatment.

Months later I began to have difficulty breathing and swallowing. I resumed taking Imuran® and underwent what was to be a two week plasmapherisis treatment. One week into the treatment I caught the flu and the fever quickly undid all the good effects of plasmapherisis. This was a particularly low point for me. But I persevered and again became symptom free. This time I reduced the prescribed dosage of the medication and no longer experienced side effects. I remained stable for many years.

Nevertheless, at a certain point in time I felt it necessary to discontinue Imuran®. I had a bout of shingles and knew I must give my body a well-deserved break from immunosuppressant drugs. My doctor and I agreed that I would switch to IVIG treatments. I responded positively to an intensive three day infusion and continued comfortably with a once every three week treatment.

Two years later I underwent an unrelated surgery that seriously exacerbated my ocular symptoms. In addition to experiencing acute double vision, I could barely lift my eyelids. The IVIG treatments were helpful for generalized MG but ineffective in relieving my eyes. Even Mestinon® didn't work!

I was deeply discouraged – this setback felt never-ending. Once again I chanted to break through this impasse. I decided to pursue the more holistic therapies - homeopathy, osteopathy, naturopathy, chiropractic, acupuncture and psychologist. I also had all my amalgam (mercury) fillings changed.

It took seven years, but today my eyes are wide open and I am in better health than I can ever remember. I am enjoying a full remission. I continue to take an IVIG treatment once every five to six weeks. I have started to hike in the summer and to snowshoe in the winter. To my surprise, I continue to improve both in endurance and skill. I feel, at age fifty-two, that I am more vital and healthier than ever.

My neurologist recently referred to me as someone who has been through it all and won. It is my firm belief that with my Buddhist practice, I have been better able to carry the disease. During my years with MG, I never stopped working or contributing to my community. And most importantly, I have not suffered - even during the hard times - as much as I could have. I am proud to say that although I have myasthenia gravis – it doesn't have me.

## PATIENT "G":

"G" is a female patient who began having MG symptoms when she was in her late teens. She is now in her mid 60's. She has autoimmune MG which was diagnosed with a Tensilon® test and repetitive nerve stimulation.

Her first symptoms were double vision, drooping eyelids and weakness of her vocal chords. It took six years from the time she sought medical help until she received the correct diagnosis. In those six years she saw about eight physicians. Her MG initially was misdiagnosed as hypothyroidism or hypoglycemia, and it was implied that her illness was psychiatric in origin. She says that she still fears that doctors will think of her as a hypochondriac. In addition to her MG she has arthritis and has been diabetic since the mid 1980's.

**SYMPTOMS:** Symptoms "G" has experienced include: Droopy lids, an inability to open her eyes, double vision, a weak smile, speech, chewing and swallowing difficulties, difficulty breathing, choking on her own secretions, weak neck and shoulder muscles, which led to an inability to support her head and difficulty holding her arms above her head. Weak arms and hands made it hard to maintain a grip or sustain activity. She also found it hard to difficult to sit in an unsupported position, rise from a chair alone, walk unassisted or climb stairs. She has experienced generalized fatigue and depression.

**TREATMENTS:** She received Mestinon® and Imuran® as treatment. Both were very effective at first. Mestinon® came first and was used exclusively for 30 years, then Imuran® was very effective, especially with swallowing problems and double vision. After using Imuran® alone for seven years she added Mestinon® because of extreme leg and arm weakness. She now takes 50 mg. of Imuran® twice daily and 60 mg. of Mestinon® three times daily.

**CURRENT LEVEL OF SYMPTOMS:** Currently she rarely experiences profound weakness, but has moderate weakness which leaves her unable to carry on with her activities from one to three days of the month and has mild weakness daily. Treatment has reduced the severity of her symptoms by 50 - 70%.

**LEVEL OF SUPPORT:** Her medical care has been supportive only in the last few years. When she was first diagnosed she was given Mestinon® and told to find the level that worked best and was given atropine to take in case she overdosed.

## PATIENT "W":

"W" is a female patient whose had double vision as her first symptom at age 39. She is now in her early 60s. She was diagnosed with a Tensilon® test, chest X-ray and CAT scan. She is seronegative. It was 16 years from the time she first sought medical help until she finally received the correct diagnosis. She saw at least 12 physicians during the diagnostic process. Her MG was initially misdiagnosed as lazy eye, anorexia and depression.

She has noticed that illness or infection (the flu etc.), stress, too little or too much sleep, getting overheated, certain antibiotics, muscle relaxants and perfumes can all make her weakness worse.

**SYMPTOMS:** She has experienced almost all the recognized MG symptoms, including nystagmus, facial weakness, nasal speech and difficulties with breathing, choking, chewing and swallowing. Weak neck muscles left her unable to support her head, weak shoulder muscles have made it difficult to hold her arms above her head. Weak hands and arms have made it hard to sustain activity and maintain her grip. She's found it difficult to walk up a ramp or climb stairs, has generalized fatigue, mental lethargy, pain and depression.

**TREATMENTS:** Mestinon®, Prostigmine®, Cytoxan® and IVIG infusion were of no help, but Prednisone®, Imuran®, CellCept® and plasmapheresis have all been effective at reducing her symptoms. Currently she takes CellCept®.

**CURRENT LEVEL OF SYMPTOMS:** She still experiences severe weakness daily, along with moderate and mild weakness. She feels that treatment has reduced the severity of her symptoms by 50%. She was included in discussions about her treatment and her care since being diagnosed has been supportive.

**"W's" STORY:** In 1980, at the age of 39, I experienced sudden double vision. Specialists told me that I had a lazy eye. This continued on and off with no benefit from the exercises they asked me to do. In 1982 I began having problems with chewing and choking and went from 110 lbs to 81 lbs. I was sent from physician to physician and told, among other things, it was nerves, depression, a digestive problem and finally that I was anorexic and "needed to get a life". A very respected neurologist made this comment to my husband and me

By this time I was convinced that it was all in my head. I pushed on working full time and began noticing my voice sounding strange. I blamed that on the problems with my throat which were caused by the problem with my head! I became weaker and started having problems with breathing and sleeping.

I reduced my working hours, thinking I needed rest. By the time I finally quit working in 1993, I could barely be understood and was mentally and physically exhausted. During the next three years, I went from internist to ear, nose and throat (ENT) specialist to speech therapy taking a variety of medications along the way. Though the speech therapist was a friend who had MG (not bulbar though) she did not recognize my symptoms.

In 1996, an ENT suggested I see a throat specialist in another teaching facility. This specialist suspected MG and requested a consult with the neurology department. They administered Tensilon® and a miracle occurred. I could speak clearly for a few minutes. After sixteen years and seeing over a dozen physicians we finally had a diagnosis. I wasn't neurotic after all !!

Immediately we started Mestinon® and learned that I am in the small percentage that cannot tolerate it. I have tried it four times since and get violently ill. I tried five IVIG treatments with no benefit. I have also learned that I am seronegative and may not respond to normal MG treatments the way that seropositive patients do.

In December of 1996 I was admitted to hospital and started Imuran® and prednisone along with 14 plasmapheresis treatments. We saw consistent improvement and by January 1, 2000 I had weaned off the prednisone and was taking only Imuran®. I had gained 60 lbs., but was so much improved. In 2002, my physician suggested we switch from Imuran® to CellCept® and I continued to remain stable. Not my old self and unable to return to work, but definitely better!

Last year was especially stressful for our family and I noticed my voice and breathing becoming a problem again. We increased the dosage of CellCept® and tried Cytoxan® with no benefit. I probably will redo the plasmapheresis and switch back to Imuran® and even take Prednisone® again if necessary.

The neurologist said when I was diagnosed, "If you have to have a neurological disease, this is the one to have, because there are treatments available." The great news is that since I have been diagnosed more treatments have become available and current research is very promising.

Having experienced symptoms for such a long time before diagnosis I wanted to become active in the local MG chapter. I especially wanted to help get information out to medical personnel and to help others get through the first shock of hearing a diagnosis that seemed like the end of the world. I had been employed all my life and felt so useless and non-productive just sitting at home.

When our daughter went back to work after the birth of our first granddaughter I asked if I could try to provide daycare for her. When one door closes one opens and she has been more than a blessing. I would have missed so much if my life had not taken this turn. She is 14 now and another little four-year-old granddaughter has stepped into her slot. Where I once thought my social life was over, I am now filling my days with a retired husband, grandchildren and volunteering for the MG chapter. Through our chapter and support groups I have met so many fantastic people with tremendous outlooks and positive lifestyles. It just reinforces how amazingly we redirect ourselves and continue on.

## PATIENT "D":

"D" is a female patient who began having MG symptoms when she was 37. She is now in her early 50s. She was diagnosed by EMG, RNS, a Tensilon® test and has anti-AChR antibodies. Her first symptom was ptosis of her left eyelid. It was seven weeks from the time she sought medical help until she received her diagnosis. She saw two physicians during the diagnostic process.

SYMPTOMS: She has experienced the full range of MG symptoms, from droopy lids and an inability to open her eyes, speaking, chewing and swallowing difficulties to respiratory crisis. She has required intubation and mechanical assistance with breathing numerous times. She uses a cane or walker but cannot walk long distances. She also experiences generalized fatigue, mental lethargy, pain and some depression.

Illness or infection, stress, too little sleep, getting overheated, menstruation and medications such as antibiotics and muscle relaxants have caused "D's" symptoms to become temporarily worse.

**TREATMENTS:** Treatments "D" has received have included Mestinon®, Prednisone® and Prostigmine®, all of which were helpful, but not as effective as plasmapherisis and Cyclosporin A®.

**CURRENT LEVEL OF SYMPTOMS:** "D" now has generalized profound weakness three or fewer days a year, moderate weakness from one to three days a month, and mild weakness during which she carries on activity with some difficulty three to six days of the week. She feels treatment and management strategies have reduced the severity of her symptoms by 75%.

**AVAILABILITY OF MG INFORMATION:** "D's" physicians gave her the information she needed during the diagnostic process and treatment. They also gave her information about MG support groups. Her medical care has been very supportive. She was included in discussions about treatment. She considers herself lucky to have a constant, caring physician.

**"D's" STORY:** "I've had MG for 16 years. I've undergone two MG crises and respiratory failure in 1997. I had squamous cell carcinoma in 1992. I had my left tonsil removed and underwent 38 radiation treatments. I think the high doses of steroids caused my diabetes and osteoporosis. I have high blood pressure, asthma, chronic laryngeal stenosis, migraines and elevated cholesterol. I've had several bouts of pneumonia and been intubated so often that I now have a permanent tracheotomy.

Shortly after I had to stop working I took some quilting classes. Quilting has proved to be a Godsend and and seems to pull me back to active status. My work now isn't as good as in the beginning but it keeps me mentally challenged. I also try to walk at least 15 minutes twice a day. The activity made a noticeable improvement. The latest X-ray of my hip replacement showed that the bone had completely mended, which was a surprise to my doctor.

When I'm depressed I give myself permission to be *pitiful,* but only for three days! During that time I write my feelings down. On day four I make myself do at least one project to get me going. In a week or so I read my letters to me - then shred the letters, as it's time to move on.

I'm blessed to have a loving and supportive husband who's hung with me through the ups and downs. My parents and my in-laws have been there to help however they could. We've learned in the last 16 years when we buy something we want then we always end up with a large medical bill or house repair soon after. It's become a joke as it always happens. We find humor wherever we can! It'll keep you going.

## AUTOIMMUNE OCULAR MG

### PATIENT "T":

"T" is a 52-year-old male patient who began having MG symptoms at age 48. His first symptom was double vision. It was four years from when he sought medical help until he received his diagnosis. He saw "about five" physicians during the diagnostic process. His symptoms were initially misdiagnosed as psychosomatic or psychiatric in nature. He had the RNS and Tensilon® tests.

**SYMPTOMS:** "T" has experienced droopy lids, an inability to open his eyes, double vision, wandering or bouncing eye, swallowing problems and depression.

**TREATMENTS:** He has taken Mestinon®, Mytelase® and Prostigmine® (all of questionable benefit), and Prednisone®. Currently he takes only Prednisone®, which controls his symptoms completely.

**AVAILABILITY OF MG INFORMATION:** He says he was only told what medications to take.

**LEVEL OF SUPPORT:** "T" says, "When I was having double vision my family doctor referred me to various other doctors, eye, ear, nose and throat specialist, and a psychiatrist - but never to a neurologist. A neurologist was suggested to me by a personal friend who was a doctor.

## CONGENITAL MYASTHENIC SYNDROMES

## FAMILIAL LIMB-GIRDLE MYASTHENIA

The following three patients are a sister and two brothers, all affected with familial limb-girdle myasthenia. We begin with the sister's story.

### A SHORT STORY ABOUT A LONG ROAD TO DIAGNOSIS:

"Fatigue and muscle weakness sneaked into my life when I was in sixth grade. At our little, four-room, brick building in Maryland, several grades were bundled into one classroom. As the school grew, the sixth grade class moved onto the stage of the school's auditorium. The few steps leading to that stage became gradually more difficult to climb as the year went on, signaling the beginning of a different life for me.

On the playground, running the bases on the softball diamond became difficult, then impossible. I could still swing the bat and hit the ball, though, so someone else in my class would run the bases for me. No questions asked.

Ours was a very small community and most kids walked to school. The school playground was the neighborhood playground, year round and the Little League baseball teams played there. My little brother, ("B") four years younger than I, was worse at running the bases than I was. The coach put him in the outfield where he wouldn't get battered by a stray line drive. Nobody ever questioned his physical shortcomings, perhaps because he spoke with a stammer and squinted through a blind eye. His fatigue and weakness, in other's minds, were probably wrapped up with the blind eye and the speech impediment.

I can only guess what my parents must have thought about "B" and me. The youngest boy, "C", was a kid of normal strength. Our parents were very caring people and good providers who would drive us to the doctor at the first hint of a cold. Why they never questioned our developing disabilities is still a mystery to me. My mother said we were lazy, and I believed her. I also believed in *spring fever*. As the weather warmed up, my arms and legs slowed down.

School was my life. I walked there, then home and back during lunch. It even had a roller rink, where some of us would go on the weekend. But, skating eventually went the way of softball. About as soon as I made some progress in roller skating I had to quit because my strength was starting to fail me.

After graduating from the sixth grade, we took the bus to Arundel Junior-Senior High School. In my 12 years I had never seen so many people in one place, not even so many people in one grade. My friends from grade school were no longer my classmates.

Rapid fatigue and muscle weakness would no longer simply insinuate itself into my life. With my first Physical Education class it crashed head-on into me. No one had ever asked me before to run laps or shoot a basketball. At that time I could still get up from a sitting position on the floor, but most exercises requiring me to use my shoulders or legs were impossible to perform. I wasn't aware of these shortcomings before PE classes. Because I tried my best and was a very good student, academically, my teacher realized that I was not faking it and let me go by. Again, no questions asked.

Over the next three years, all my PE teachers noted that something was wrong with my balance or coordination, and remarked about it on my report cards. No questions asked at home. None by the school bus driver, either, who saw that I struggled getting up the steps into the bus with a load of books in my arms. He would simply get up and kindly give me a hand up the steps.

One of the most humiliating experiences of my life was having the 10th grade PE teacher bring me out of the ranks and try to make me do a thrust-squat. I could get down to the floor, but I could never thrust my legs backward. She asked me why I thought I couldn't do it, and I ventured that maybe I was too heavy. That's what it felt like to me, anyway. Then out of the ranks she pulled another girl, this time one who was tall and heavy. She made us both weigh ourselves, then had the big girl do repeated squat thrusts.

Having proven that my weight was not the problem, the teacher then asked me to do a squat thrust again. I tried it, couldn't do it, then suffered even more indignities when I offered that my arms felt too weak to hold me up. She made me push against her outstretched arms which made me dance around the gym floor like a rubbery marionette. She told me that I'd better know how to do it when I came back on Monday. I was so confused that I spent the weekend trying to master the squat thrust, hoping that there was some trick to it that I was missing.

The following Monday morning I marched into the guidance counselor's office and told him my story. He allowed me to substitute choral music for physical education until I left school. He never asked if I had ever seen a doctor.

Life was beautiful again without PE. My grades were good and I enjoyed choral singing enormously. I never gave my physical strength or fatigue much thought after that until the end of my sophomore year when I contracted a virus of some kind. It flattened me for a long time. I was at home sick for at least two weeks with a fever. For an even longer time afterward I was very conscious of my weak muscles. I lost about 20 pounds and was very pale. Stepping up onto an ordinary sidewalk became very difficult. At the time I was taking music lessons on the piano and the accordion, the latter being tantamount to holding half a piano in your lap. Accordion lessons came to a stop because I couldn't pull the bellows back and forth.

I married very young and had three babies. Pregnancy was difficult only in the first trimester and after the birth. I felt very tired and weak and had trouble carrying and handling my babies, but I still thought I had spring fever or something.

While I was living in my love bubble and having babies, my brother, "B", was getting attention at school because of his fatigue and muscle weakness. He was able to hide his falls and other difficulties because his friends would come to his rescue, pick him up from the ground, carry books for him and assist him onto the school bus. In high school, PE was "B"'s hulking monster, as it had been mine. My parents finally took him to our family doctor who saw him several times and did some blood work before sending him off to Johns Hopkins Hospital in Baltimore.

At "B"'s first appointment at Johns Hopkins, the physician gave him a neurological work-up, observing that he had fatigue and muscle weakness, but no ocular or bulbar involvement. He sent my brother home without a diagnosis, to return in six months, so that any changes in his condition could be observed. But before sending him off, the doctor asked: "Does anyone else in your have family have muscle weakness?" For the first time in my life somebody's medical finger was pointing at me.

In May, 1963, just after the birth of my second child, I accompanied "B" to Johns Hopkins Hospital. We were examined, and told to return in six months. The happy outcome of that visit is that I had a file at Johns Hopkins and an appointment to return.

Not long before that November appointment my car was rear-ended, resulting in a slight sprain of my neck. Because my old family doctor was not available, I went to somebody else's old family doctor whom I had never met before. This diminutive man with coke-bottle-like eyeglass lenses gave me a brief neuro work-up, testing reflexes and such.

Then he asked me to lift my legs. I couldn't do that lying flat on my back. "What! Are you paralyzed?" he asked. I simply told him what I knew. My legs and arms were weak. They had almost always been that way. He scowled at me and asked me to perform a couple of other small tasks like getting up from a chair, holding out my arms, the usual stuff. Then he sang these words to me: "I have an idea of what your problem is. Would you like to come back in a week for a test?" I would have crawled back over broken glass to hear more of that music.

**MAKING THE SHORT STORY EVEN LONGER:** The test I was given a week later was an injection of Prostigmine® or neostigmine. It allowed me to lift my arms and legs better than I ever remembered. This family doctor had studied MG somewhere and guessed at the diagnosis. He wrote "Myasthenia Gravis" on the back of his business card. I took it with me to Johns Hopkins on our next appointment.

"B" and I were admitted to Johns Hopkins Hospital for 10 days of testing. Our neurologist there, Dr. Michael McQuillen, invented a term for our condition: *Familial Limb-Girdle Myasthenia*. That was in 1963. Not much was known then about MG. "B" and I enjoyed significant improvement from the Mestinon we were prescribed. Our MG was fairly stable for years after that. Our brother, "C", started showing symptoms much later.

From 1966 through 1972 my strength stayed relatively stable. I took my degree in French. In 1974 I enjoyed a great improvement in my strength which lasted almost two years. I rode a bicycle for short distances and was able to lift dishes into the cabinets and do my hair without much trouble. 1975 was a very good year for me. I took my kids to France, and enrolled in the university to study French language and culture.

In 1976 I got much weaker. I was prescribed large doses of Prednisone®. My strength improved somewhat, but not enough to warrant the steroids. (Later tests determined that all three of us are AChR antibody negative.) However I was able to work full time and care for my kids and house. In the late '80s I began to get gradually weaker until 1988 when I began to fall more often and began having more difficulty negotiating stairs, lifting my arms, etc.

It was then that I called Johns Hopkins and begged them to tell me they had something new in their bag of tricks to treat MG. My timing was good. I was admitted to a study of 3, 4 – diaminopyridine (DAP) at the Mayo Clinic. I have been taking DAP since 1989 and so have both of my brothers. Eventually the three of us were accepted into the DAP study at Duke University in Durham, NC. My brothers and I are now seen at Penn/Hershey Medical Center in Hershey, PA.

Over the 50 years more or less that I have had MG, my illness has been gradually progressive with occasional periods of improvements. It is impossible to determine the cause of the ebbs and flows of strength and weakness. Sometimes it appears to be related to stress and sadness, but not always. Certainly an entire day of fatigue and weakness will follow a day of stress and exertion, but this does not explain the prolonged exacerbations. Improvement in strength can happen just as unexpectedly. I remember a hot day in July a few years ago when my husband and I were exploring a Civil War battleground in Virginia on our way to Duke University. I started walking up a hill and with every step I took up I felt stronger. This continued for weeks, then months, and I enjoyed gardening, weight loss, and high spirits.

The key to coping with this physical and psychological uncertainty is to find a form of distraction that is restful to your body and mind. I escape with a movie. This allows me to park my body and my mind for an hour and a half and feel refreshed afterwards. Reading, letter writing or computer play might work for others. "Allow" is the key word here. As myasthenics we tend to over-cope instead of giving ourselves what we need: rest.

## BROTHER "B":

"B" began having symptoms of myasthenia at age 12, but was slower than average physically all through childhood. He was diagnosed while in his teens and is now in his mid-50s. Tests used in the diagnostic process were EMG and RNS. His first myasthenic symptom was falling down. It was four years from when "B" first sought medical help until he received a diagnosis, and he says he saw "lots of interns". He says no one ever suggested his symptoms were psychosomatic or psychiatric, but it was suggested that he was lazy. Specific triggers which seem to make his symptoms worse include illness or infection (the flu etc.), stress, getting overheated, drinking alcohol, and some foods, MSG is one.

SYMPTOMS: "B's" symptoms include weak neck and shoulder muscles and weak arms. He has difficulty sustaining activity, climbing stairs and suffers from generalized fatigue. He sometimes uses a mobility device but can walk a quarter of a mile on good day.

TREATMENTS: Mestinon® and DAP.

CURRENT LEVEL OF SYMPTOMS: "B" carries on daily activities with some difficulty. Treatment has reduced the severity of his symptoms by 50%, but his level of weakness varies hourly.

AVAILABILITY OF MG INFORMATION: His physicians gave him the information he needed during the diagnostic process and included him in the decision-making process. His medical care has been supportive.

"B's" COMMENTS: "My siblings and I treat MG with a touch of humor. We are able to look at the falls and problems associated with MG and laugh at them or just say sh*t when we fall or have a bad time.

I live in Annapolis, Maryland, the home of the U.S. Naval Academy. One Sunday morning I went to get my wife some bagels. I was parked at the front door of the shop. Several naval cadets were having a meal at the glass store front facing my car. I left the shop and fell behind my car. The cadets didn't come to help me. Two men walking down the sidewalk helped me up. After shaking their hands and saying thank you, I turned to the cadets in the window, took a bow, got into my car and went home.

My sister and I have had MG for so long that it is our norm. We love the good days and realize the bad days will pass and as persons with MG, if we want it done, we better do it on the first try.

## BROTHER "C":

"C" began having MG symptoms when he was 29 years old. He is now in his mid-50s. Tests used during the diagnostic process were EMG, RNS, Tensilon®, anti-AChR antibody, chest X-ray and CT scan.

In the mid 1960s, when "C" was about 14 years old, his brother and sister were diagnosed with myasthenia, but he had no symptoms at that time. He went on to lead a normal life, served in the military, married and had two children. In 1978 he noticed that it was more difficult for him to carry his second child around than it had been with the first child. His shoes felt as if they had weights in them, and when he carried groceries the bags would slip lower and lower as his arm muscles tired. He was working jobs which required physical strength, first driving a truck and then as a welder.

In late 1980 he sought medical help at Johns Hopkins Hospital, where he was diagnosed with congenital myasthenia. His symptoms responded to Mestinon®, and he continued to lead a normal life. He was aware of the family history of congenital myasthenia when he sought medical help. He saw three physicians during the diagnostic process and received his diagnosis in two months.

**SYMPTOMS:** "C" has experienced the following symptoms: Difficulty chewing, weak shoulder muscles, difficult to hold arms above head, weak arms, hard to sustain activity, weak hands, hard to maintain grip, difficulty breathing (one time), difficulty rising from a chair unassisted, difficulty walking unassisted (uses a mobility device), can walk *very short* distance unassisted, difficulty walking up a ramp, difficulty climbing stairs, foot drop, generalized fatigue, pain in calves of legs, foot cramps and depression.

He notes that illness or infection, stress, too much or too little sleep, getting chilled or overheated, drinking alcohol, medications such as antibiotics and muscle relaxants and emotional extremes, both positive and negative, can trigger weakness.

**TREATMENTS:**    He takes Mestinon® (very effective), Prostigmine®, and 100 mg. of DAP daily (highly effective).

**CURRENT LEVEL OF SYMPTOMS:** "C" currently has generalized profound weakness one to three days a week, moderate weakness which leaves him unable to carry on with his activities three to six days a week, and mild weakness during which he can carry on with his activities with some difficulty daily. One to three days of the month he has only very mild weakness. Treatment has reduced the severity of his symptoms by 50%.

**AVAILABILITY OF MG INFORMATION:** "C's" physicians provided him the information he needed during the diagnostic and treatment process. He was told about the MGFA and made aware of their services. His medical care was mostly supportive.

**"C's" Comments:** "I was taking one tablet of Mestinon® daily and functioned well until around October of 1993. At that time I noticed more weakness and fatigue. It progressed until I had to quit work as a truck driver and go on disability. I was then accepted into the DAP study at Duke University. After 10 days of tests I was put on DAP and Mestinon®. It helped a lot but I still felt weak a lot of the time and was fatigued, and I still fell a lot. On my own I increased my dose of Mestinon® to 60 mg. (one tablet) every four to five hours. It worked out a lot better and that is what I am taking now.

Since being diagnosed things have occurred that are typical of those with MG, but in my case I have good days and bad days. One day I can feel great and do a lot, others I can't seem to do anything.

There are ups and downs with the medications. Sometimes it seems it takes forever for them to kick in, and other times they take effect almost instantly.

My biggest problem is getting up from low chairs, or getting up from the ground after falling. I hate going up stairs. Escalators scare me because of the movement and having to be in step getting on or off. When getting groceries I always use a cart for support, even for one item. Occasionally I use the electric cart.

From February 2002 to August 2003 I attended a school for people with disabilities and got a degree in computer-aided drafting. This school was 13 acres under one roof. The staff arranged for me to get my own electric cart because of the distance from class to class.

I now realize that I have had MG since birth. In 1976 I was banged up in an auto accident, but not seriously hurt. About six months later I started noticing symptoms. I fell in 1992, fracturing a vertebrae, and in six - eight months my symptoms grew worse, eventually forcing me to quit work and apply for disability. I believe the auto accident caused my MG to come out of remission and settle at a certain level, then a second trauma caused the symptoms to become worse and put me where I am today.

All the doctors I have seen over the years have been very supportive, except for my family doctor. When I was applying for disability benefits he would not support my claim. His comment was that if I could walk into his office I was not handicapped.

## INDIVIDUAL PATIENT'S COMMENTS

Looking back at these comments, I see and hear my friends again. All were members of our local MG support group. These were not negative people. They were full of laughter, jokes and fun. They lived with a sense of gratitude and joy and did not dwell on their illness. Yet when given opportunity to express their deepest feelings, emotional pain and a sense of betrayal often surfaced.

When MG patients seek treatment they often know more about MG, its treatment and potential complications than do the physicians treating them. It can be deeply upsetting when a physician will not believe them or listen to them. Denying that MG patients face problems with diagnosis, medical care, relationships and physical weakness is dishonest.

In the past 20 years I have met many MG patients. Most of them manage to live fairly normal lives. Most submerge their worries and fears and drag out the fortitude on a daily basis, but they remain vividly human, self-doubting, and profoundly sensitive to the attitudes of those around them. The comments which follow were made by friends with MG, and I am grateful that they shared them with us.

### COMMENTS ON EARLY SYMPTOMS

- I started by having trouble with my arms. I couldn't comb my hair at times or lift things. No one suspected MG for years because I was strong otherwise.
- I was swimming and found I couldn't move my arms or legs. The lifeguard pulled me out of the water and called an ambulance but by the time they arrived I was able to move again and everyone got mad at me.
- I thought I was going blind. I didn't realize I couldn't open my eyes more than a slit. I went to an ophthalmologist but he said my eyes were fine. On the way home from his office my eyes closed and I couldn't open them. I was stopped at a red light and I was unable to see to drive the car.
- I was out to dinner with a friend who is a doctor. He noticed my eyelid drooping and that I was having trouble chewing and asked me to to see a specialist he knew right away.
- I had been tired for a long time but one night I went out to walk the dog and I fell down and couldn't get up. My legs felt like stone.

## ON DOCTORS AND THE DIAGNOSTIC PROCESS

- The last doctor I saw was very supportive. The others had made me feel like some kind of deviant. He was much more thorough than the others. At one point he said that if it (my MG) wasn't 'textbook' the likes of doctors "A" and "B" would never see it. I suppose that wasn't the kind of thing one doctor should say about another but it made me feel normal and human again.
- My own doctor didn't know too much about it (MG) but said he would find out and we would work at it together. I really respect him for that.
- I was in crisis in the hospital and couldn't speak, so I wrote my questions in a little notebook. When the doctor came I handed him the notebook. He threw it at me and growled, "I don't have time for this," and stomped out.
- When my doctor told me I had MG I started to cry. He was so kind. He said I have a relatively mild case and I could lead a full life even with MG. He showed so much confidence in me that I was able to deal with it.
- The doctor told my parents I was just looking for attention (patient was 10 years old). He said if I fell down crossing the highway again just to leave me there and I would get up before a car hit me.
- My neurologist had seen me for several years. One day he handed me a jump rope and told me if I wanted to I could jump it, that I was just looking for sympathy.
- I had been sent to a neurologist every year for four years. I got worse and worse but he always sent me to a psychiatrist. Each time the psychiatrist told him that I'm not crazy, I'm sick. Finally I went home to Europe because I expected to die. The pilot radioed to have an ambulance meet the plane. Within hours they told me that I had MG. I had a thymectomy the next day. My thymus was bigger than my surgeon's hand. I was 10 months in hospital.
- I already had a neurologist because I have seizures. I went right away when my eyes started to droop. He examined me and told me he thought I had MG.
- My husband asked the neurologist a question and the doctor said, "Who do you think you are? You're not a physician." During another appointment this doctor just got up and walked out of the room while I was talking. The next time I saw him I tried to talk quickly so as not to take up too much time and he asked, "Are you always this anxious?"

- The neurologist wouldn't answer my questions. He handed me a prescription for prednisone and said he would take care of me. He didn't tell me it might make me worse.
- I had several EMGs over a period of years, all with negative results. Finally an Internist did a Tensilon® test on me and the difference was striking.

## ON LIVING WITH MG

- I get angry. I think, *Why me?* I'd never been sick. I always was the one who took care of everyone else.
- I had to learn to pace myself. I have to stop and rest before I get too tired.
- I've learned to do my heavier work early in the day, lighter things in the afternoon and plan to do nothing in the evening because I've had it by then.
- I stayed in the house for years. I didn't see anyone. I thought it might be catching. I always take a friend or a family member when I go out. I stagger, fall, get slurred speech. People have thought I was drunk in the past and that's humiliating.
- I have good days and bad days. I feel so happy on my good days, but I really hate it when I get a bad day and can't do anything.
- I won't let it rule my life. I push myself to do what I want to do, even though I put myself in the hospital sometimes.
- I feel so guilty asking for help from my family. I'm supposed to take care of my children, not the other way around.
- I feel like it's everyone's responsibility to do what they can to help around the house. I do as much as I can and they do the rest.
- It isolates you. People see you don't feel well or you can't smile or talk and they feel sorry for you but they don't want to be with you very much.
- The most important thing for me is not to let myself get mentally down. Sometimes I'm too weak to do much but if I'm a little better I'll write letters or figure out how to organize something. I took up some new quiet hobbies.
- I've learned If I don't feel strong I'm better resting than trying to push myself. If I keep pushing I just will get worse. If I rest I often feel better.
- I'm usually O.K. - until I see somebody on the TV running up a hill or dancing or playing with their children. Catch me on a bad day and that can start the tears.

## ON HOSPITAL CARE

- Sometimes you have to be really firm and refuse to do what they want you to do, when you know it's dangerous for you.
- The pheresis team was just great. They were knowledgeable about MG and understood how frightened I was.
- The nurses were terrific. They came and said, "You know MG and your own body. How do we take care of you?"
- You have to be careful if you're seen by a doctor other than your own. Twice I've had a crisis after being prescribed drugs that MG patients shouldn't take.
- The nurses were reluctant to leave my Mestinon® at the bedside, but I told them my doctor trusts me to take it without supervision at home, why can't I take it here? I need it right on time, not 20 minutes late. They decided that it was a reasonable request.
- No matter what I said they wouldn't leave my Mestinon® with me. They were always late and when I complained the nurse said that half an hour couldn't possibly make any difference.
- My own doctor was on holidays when I had an accident and had to have surgery. Although my family talked to the doctor in charge they gave me injections of morphine and discontinued my Mestinon®. I went into crisis. Finally my daughter literally kidnapped me from the hospital and took me home.

## ON FAMILY AND FRIENDS

- My family and friends have been great. They say, "Do you need a pill? Do you need a rest?"
- My daughter gets angry when I can't do her laundry. If I tell her I don't feel well, she says she's tired of that excuse.
- My parents just don't want to accept that anything could be wrong with me. They pretend not to see my symptoms and they turn away if I try to talk to them.
- My husband left me when I got sick.

## NOTES:

# GLOSSARY

**Acetylcholine (ACh):** A chemical produced by the body, which acts a a transmitter of nerve impulses.

**Acetylcholine receptor (AChR):** A structure located on the folds of the neuromuscular junction which acts as a receiver for ACh; the site of the immune system attack in autoimmune based MG.

**Acetylcholinesterase:** An enzyme produced by the body which acts as an antagonist to acetylcholine, causing it to break down.

**AChR antibodies – (anti-AChR antibodies):** Defensive proteins, produced by the immune system, which attack the AChR.

**Adrenal glands:** A set of paired organs that sit on top of the kidneys, producing adrenalin, hydrocortisone and aldosterone, hormones which control mineral levels, stress reactions and energy metabolism among other things.

**Angina:** Heart muscle pain which comes with exertion.

**Anaphylactic shock:** Severe allergic reaction which may include skin redness, itching, water accumulation in tissues, swelling, drop in blood pressure, spasm of the lungs and shock.

**Anemia:** A condition in which there are too few red blood cells.

**Anesthesiologist:** A medical doctor who has specialized in the administration and control of anesthesia during surgery.

**Antibodies:** Specialized proteins which form the body's defense system against bacterial and viral invasion. For reasons that are still poorly understood, the body sometimes produces antibodies that attack its own tissues and organs (autoantibodies).

**Anticholinesterases:** Medications which prolong the action of acetylcholine by blocking its antagonist, acetylcholinesterase.

**Apgar score:** A test done one minute and five minutes after birth to determine a newborn baby's physical health. Scoring is based on five factors that rate how well a baby is adjusting to life outside the womb.

**Apnea:** Temporary pause in breathing.

**ARIA:** Acronym for **A**cetylcholine **R**eceptor **I**nducing **A**ctivity.

**Arthrogryposis:** The fixation of a joint in an extended or flexed position.

**Atrophy:** A condition in which muscles become smaller.

**Autoimmune disease:** A disease or disorder caused by elements of the immune system attacking some of the body's tissues or organs. Examples of immune system diseases and the organs involved are: myasthenia gravis, neuromuscular junction; Crohn's disease, digestive system; diabetes, pancreas, rheumatoid arthritis, cartilage; systemic lupus erythematosus (SLE), collagen (or connective) tissue.

**Autosomal dominant inheritance pattern:** Only one parent need carry the gene mutation. Each child has a 50% chance of inheriting the disorder from the parent carrying the mutation.

**Autosomal recessive inheritance pattern:** Both parents must carry the gene mutation. Each child has a 25% chance of inheriting the mutation.

**Asymptomatic:** Without discernible symptoms.

**Basal Lamina:** A tissue in the  synaptic cleft which separates the nerve and muscle cell membranes. The basal lamina contains a protein called *agrin*. When agrin is added to a culture containing muscle cells AChRs gather and grow in the muscle membrane.

**Bulbar:** Referring to the muscles used in speaking, chewing, swallowing and breathing.

**Cartilage:** A rubbery tissue which covers joint surfaces.

**Cell nucleus:** Control center of the cell, contains the genetic information the cell needs to reproduce itself.

**Cell plasma membrane:** The cell's outside skin.

**Cholinergic crisis:** Myasthenic crisis brought on by an excess of anticholinesterase medication. Symptoms include muscle weakness and twitching, increased salivation, sweating and constricted pupils.

**Cholinergic pathways:** Parts of the nervous system that use acetylcholine as the neurotransmitter.

**Chromosomes:** Structures which contain and organize genes. Humans have 23 pairs of chromosomes in each cell, for a total of 46. Twenty-two pairs (the autosomes) are the same in males and females. Pair 23 are the sex chromosomes. These are different in males and females. Females have two copies of the X chromosome, while males have one X and one Y.

**Congenital myasthenic syndrome (CMS):** Myasthenia that is caused by an inborn defect in the neuromuscular junction. Those with congenital myasthenia do not have anti-AChR antibodies and usually develop symptoms early in childhood.

**Contraindicated:** A term used to indicate that a particular medication or type of medication should not be administered to persons with a known history of a specific disease.

**Contraindications:** Don't give this drug to patients who have the conditions listed in this section.

**Curare:** A drug derived from a South American plant, once was used to induce muscle paralysis during surgery.

**Cushingoid appearance:** The development of a round 'moon face' and weight gain following the administration of corticosteroid drugs.

**Electroencephalogram (EEG):** A test which records brain waves.

**Electromyography (EMG):** A test that measures the electrical activity in muscles. EMG used as a general term includes nerve conduction study (NCS) and repetitive nerve stimulation (RNS).

**Electrophysiological evidence:** The appearance of recognized abnormal patterns of nerve or muscle reaction during electromyography or nerve conduction tests.

**Encode:** To specify the genetic code for.

**Endplate Potential:** The temporary depolarization of the muscle membrane caused by activation of ACh receptor sites.

**Enzyme:** A protein that causes or speeds up chemical reactions in living matter.

**Exacerbation:** A period of time when symptoms of a disease become more severe.

**Exophthalmos**: Abnormal protrusion of the eyeball.

**External ophthalmoplegia:** Limitation of eye movements; the eye is unable to look up, down or inwards.

**Extraocular:** Any of six small voluntary muscles that pass between the eyeball and the orbit and control the movement of the eyeball in relation to the orbit.

**Familial myasthenia gravis (FMG):** A rare type of autoimmune MG that occurs in two or more members of the same family.

**Fulminant:** Rapid, sudden or severe.

**Gamma globulin:** One factor in the blood which acts as a defense mechanism (see antibodies).

**Genetic predisposition:** A tendency to develop a condition or disease due to genetic influences which requires one or more triggering factors to initiate.

**Genome:** Genetic information needed to replicate an entire organism, encoded in deoxyribonucleic acid (DNA), and organized into units called genes.

**Hypopnea:** Abnormally slow or especially shallow respiration.

**Hypoventilation:** Deficient ventilation of the lungs that results in reduction in the oxygen content or increase in the carbon dioxide content of the blood or both.

**Idiopathic:** Cause unknown.

**Immunoactive substance:** See antibodies, gamma globulin, immunoglobulin.

**Immunoglobulin:** A part of the body's defense system, contained in the blood (see antibodies).

**Involuntary muscle:** See smooth muscle.

**Ion channels:** Pores which pierce the cell membrane and control the flow of molecules like sodium, calcium and potassium in and out of the cell.

**Irradiation:** Treatment of malignancies or immune system disease with specific types of radiation.

**Jitter:** The variation in time between electrical signals recorded from two muscle fibers served by the same nerve. When neuromuscular transmission is impaired the time variation (recorded with SFEMG) between signals increases, creating what is called 'jitter'.

**Lambert-Eaton myasthenic syndrome (LEMS):** A condition, often accompanying small cell carcinoma of the lung, which reduces the amount of acetylcholine released at the neuromuscular junction, producing weakness similar to MG.

**Ligand-gated:** Permitting or blocking passage through an ion channel in response to a chemical stimulus.

**Systemic Lupus erythematosus: (SLE)** See Autoimmune disease.

**Motor nerves:** Nerves which carry nerve signals to muscle, and are involved in movement.

**Mutation:** A permanent change in a gene which alters the physical trait carried by the gene.

**Myopathy:** Muscle disease.

**Nasogastric feeding tube:** A flexible tybe which is inserted through the nose, down the throat and into the stomach. The patient can be fed a nutrient solution through the tube.

**Neonatal myasthenia gravis (NMG):** A temporary form of MG found in the newborn child (the neonate) of a myasthenic mother.

**Neural:** Pertaining to the nerves.

**Neuromuscular:** Used to described the neuromuscular junction, or diseases which involve both the nerves and /or muscles.

**Neuromuscular blocker:** Any chemical substance that interferes with the transmission of impulses through the neuromuscular junction.

**Neuromuscular junction:** The junction of the structures of the motor nerve axon and the muscle membrane, including the synaptic cleft, basal lamina, AChR sites and endplates.

**Neurotransmitter:** Any chemical that results in the sending of nerve signals across a synapse.

**Neuromuscular transmission:** The passing of the impulse from the nerve ending to the muscle via the neuromuscular junction.

**Nystagmus:** Involuntary, rhythmic movement of the eye, side-to-side, up and down, around or mixed.

**Ocular:** Having to do with the eyes.

**Oropharyngeal:** Relating to the mouth and soft palate.

**Pancytopenia:** A marked reduction in the number of red and white blood cells, and in the number of platelets.

**Plasmapheresis - Plasma exchange: (PE or PLEx)** A mechanical method of removing antibodies from a patient's blood.

**Polycythemia:** An abnormally high red blood cell count.

**Polyhydramnios:** The presence of excessive amniotic fluid.

**Postural scoliosis:** An abnormal curve in the spine which develops as weak trunk muscles tire with standing or sitting.

**Ptosis:** Drooping of the upper eyelid.

**Rapid turnover (RTO):** Acetylcholine receptor sites which are short-lived and are quickly replaced.

**Remission:** A period of time in which symptoms go away, may be temporary or permanent.

**Respiratory depression or failure:** Decreased ability to breathe or an inability to breathe adequately

**Seronegative:** Having a negative reaction to a test for the presence of an antibody.

**Seronegative myasthenia gravis:** A form of MG in which the patients do not have anti-AChR antibodies, considered by some neurologists to be a variant form of the disease due to yet undiscovered antibodies.

**Siblings:** Brothers or sisters.

**Single-fiber electromyography (SFEMG):** A test designed to check for 'jitter' or blocking in a patient suspected of having MG (see 'jitter').

**Sleep apnea:** A temporary pause in breathing during sleep.

**Smooth muscle (involuntary):** Muscle we do not exert voluntary control over, such as the heart, digestive tract and uterus.

**Soft palate:** Area at the back and top of the mouth.

**Sphincter:** Ring-shaped muscles which control the outlets of the bladder and bowel.

**Sporadic:** A spontaneous genetic mutation which is not inherited.

**Stem cell:** The most primitive cells in the bone marrow, from which all blood cells grow.

**Sternum:** The breastbone.

**Striated or Skeletal muscle (voluntary):** Muscle that we have voluntary control over, such as facial and limb muscle.

**Syndrome:** A group of signs and symptoms that occur together and are typical of a particular disease or disorder.

**Thymectomy:** The surgical removal of the thymus gland.

**Thymoma:** A tumor, either benign or malignant, of the thymus gland.

**Thymus:** A butterfly-shaped nodular organ located beneath the sternum, involved in the activation of immune cells.

**Trachea:** The windpipe.

**Vesicles:** Small bulb-shaped organs at nerve endings that secrete ACh. also a small fluid-filled sac or blister.

**Voluntary muscles:** See striated or skeletal muscle.

# APPENDIX

## STRENGTH LEVEL TESTING CHART

| Date | Muscle Group Tested | # of Repetitions or Minutes Unmedicated | # of Repetitions or Minutes Medicated | Scale of 1-10 |
|------|------|------|------|------|
|  |  |  |  |  |
|  |  |  |  |  |
|  |  |  |  |  |
|  |  |  |  |  |
|  |  |  |  |  |
|  |  |  |  |  |
|  |  |  |  |  |
|  |  |  |  |  |
|  |  |  |  |  |
|  |  |  |  |  |
|  |  |  |  |  |
|  |  |  |  |  |
|  |  |  |  |  |
|  |  |  |  |  |
|  |  |  |  |  |
|  |  |  |  |  |

## PRESCRIBED MEDICATIONS CHART

**NAME:**

| | |
|---|---|
| *Medication* | |
| Date began | |
| Dosage / schedule | |
| Benefits | |
| Side Effects | |
| *Medication* | |
| Date began | |
| Dosage/schedule | |
| Benefits | |
| Side Effects | |
| *Medication* | |
| Date began | |
| Dosage/schedule | |
| Benefits | |
| Side Effects | |
| *Medication* | |
| Date began | |
| Dosage/schedule | |
| Benefits | |
| Side Effects | |
| *Medication* | |
| Date began | |
| Dosage/schedule | |
| Benefits | |
| Side Effects | |

## OVER-THE-COUNTER DRUG AND SUPPLEMENTS RECORD

**NAME:**

| | |
|---|---|
| **OTC Drug or Supplement** | |
| Dosage/schedule | |
| Date began | |
| Benefits | |
| Side Effects | |
| **OTC Drug or Supplement** | |
| Dosage/schedule | |
| Date began | |
| Benefits | |
| Side Effects | |
| **OTC Drug or Supplement** | |
| Dosage/schedule | |
| Date began | |
| Benefits | |
| Side Effects | |
| **OTC Drug or Supplement** | |
| Dosage/schedule | |
| Date began | |
| Benefits | |
| Side Effects | |

**RECORD OF PHYSICIANS' VISITS:**

**NAME:**

| | |
|---|---|
| **Physician's Name** | |
| Date | |
| Reason for Visit | |
| Outcome | |
| Tests ordered | |
| Treatment begun | |
| **Physician's Name** | |
| Date | |
| Reason for Visit | |
| Outcome | |
| Tests ordered | |
| Treatment begun | |
| **Physician's Name** | |
| Date | |
| Reason for Visit | |
| Outcome | |
| Tests ordered | |
| **Physician's Name** | |
| Date | |
| Reason for Visit | |
| Outcome | |
| Tests ordered | |
| Treatment begun | |

## RECORD OF TESTS PERFORMED:

### NAME:

| Physician's Name | |
|---|---|
| Date | |
| Reason for Test | |
| Outcome | |
| **Physician's Name** | |
| Date | |
| Reason for Test | |
| Outcome | |
| **Physician's Name** | |
| Date | |
| Reason for Test | |
| Outcome | |
| **Physician's Name** | |
| Date | |
| Reason for Test | |
| Outcome | |
| **Physician's Name** | |
| Date | |
| Reason for Test | |
| Outcome | |
| **Physician's Name** | |
| Date | |
| Reason for Test | |
| Outcome | |

**ANESTHESIA HISTORY CHART:**

**NAME:**

| | |
|---|---|
| Date | |
| Procedure | |
| Anesthetic: | |
| Dose | |
| Route (IV, Epidural, General) | |
| Side Effects: | |
| Date | |
| Procedure | |
| Anesthetic: | |
| Dose | |
| Route (IV, Epidural, General) | |
| Side Effects: | |
| Date | |
| Procedure | |
| Anesthetic: | |
| Dose | |
| Route (IV, Epidural, General) | |
| Side Effects: | |

## SOMATIZATION DISORDER CRITERIA

**SYMPTOMS:** A history of many physical complaints occurring over a period of several years, beginning before age 30. The patient seeks treatment, or suffers significant impairment in social, occupational, or other important areas of functioning. *To meet the diagnostic criteria for Somatization Disorder EACH of the following criteria must have been met.*

**FOUR PAIN SYMPTOMS:** A history of pain related to at least four different sites or functions such as headache, abdominal pain, back/joint pain, pain in the extremities, chest pain, pain in the rectum, pain during menstruation, sexual intercourse, or urination.

**TWO GASTROINTESTINAL SYMPTOMS:** A history of at least two gastrointestinal symptoms other than pain such as persistent nausea, bloating, or vomiting other than during pregnancy, diarrhea, or intolerance of several different foods.

**ONE SEXUAL SYMPTOM:** A history of at least one sexual or reproductive symptom, other than pain, such as sexual indifference, erectile or ejaculatory dysfunction, irregular menses, excessive menstrual bleeding, or vomiting throughout pregnancy.

**ONE PSEUDONEUROLOGICAL SYMPTOM:** A history of at least one symptom suggesting a neurological condition not limited to pain such as impaired coordination or balance, paralysis or localized weakness, difficulty swallowing or lump in throat, inability to speak normally, urinary retention, hallucinations, loss of touch or pain sensation, double vision, blindness, deafness, seizures; amnesia; or loss of consciousness other than fainting.

**PATIENT'S SYMPTOMS MUST FULFILL 1, 2 OR 3 BELOW:**
    1. *After appropriate investigation*, the patient's symptoms cannot be fully explained by a known general medical condition or the direct effects of a substance (e.g., drug abuse, side effects of a medication).
    2. When there is a related general medical condition, the physical complaints or resulting impairment are in excess of what would be expected from the history, physical examination, or laboratory findings
    3. The symptoms are not intentionally feigned or produced.

**HOW TO OBTAIN THE COLLIS-CURVE® TOOTHBRUSH**

http://www.colliscurve.com/

In the US: 6110 California Road, Brownsville, TX, 78521

Ph: 800-298-4818 FAX: 956-546-4818

In Canada: Phone/fax (403) 246-3302

# REFERENCES

## CHAPTER ONE:

- Alberts, B; Bray, D; Lewis, J; ct al; *Molecular Biology of the Cell* 3rd ed. New York and London: Garland Pub; 1994.
- Berg, JM; Tymoczko, JL; and Stryer, L: Biochemistry IV. Responding to Environmental Changes 33. *The Immune System*. New York: W. H. Freeman and Co.; 2002.
- Cooper, GM; *The Cell – A Molecular Approach* - 2nd ed. Sunderland (MA): Sinauer Assoc. Inc.; 2000.
- Griffiths, AJF; Miller, JH; Suzuki, DT; et al; *Introduction to Genetic Analysis* 7th ed. NYC; W. H. Freeman and Co.; 1999.
- Hoch, W; McConville J; Helms S; et al; (2001) Auto-antibodies to the receptor tyrosine kinase MuSK in patients with MG without acetylcholine receptor antibodies. Nature Medicine, 7; 365-368.
- Janeway, CA; Travers P; Walport M; Shlomchik M; *Immunobiology* 5th ed. NYC and London: Garland Pub; 2001.
- Lauralee Sherwood; *Human Physiology - From Cells to Systems* 4th ed. 2001- ISBN: 0534568262
- Lodish H; Berk A; Zipursky S; et al; *Molecular Cell Biology* 4th ed. New York: W. H. Freeman & Co.;2000.
- Lombroso PJ; Mercadante MT; *Genetics of Childhood Disorders;* XXIX Autoimmune Disorders Part Three: MG and Rasmussen's Encephalitis; J Am Acad Child Adolesc Psychiatry, 40:9,1115-1117;9:2001
- Megeath LJ; Kirber MT; Hopf C; et.al. ;Calcium-dependent maintenance of agrin-induced post-synaptic specializations. Neuroscience. 2003;122(3):659-68.
- Nicolle MW; Personal Correspondence. 2 May, 2005.
- Pestronk A; Drachman D; Antibody-Mediated Membrane Abnormalities in PM: Reduction of AChRs by IgG. *MG Biology and Treatment*, New York Academy of Sciences, Vol. 505, 1987, pp. 357-367.
- Ramsay DA; Drachman DB; Drachman RJ; et.al.; Stabilization of acetylcholine receptors at the neuromuscular synapse: the role of the nerve. Brain Res. 1992 May 29; 581(2):198-207.

· Riddle, DL; Blumenthal T; Meyer B J; et al; eds. *C elegans II.* Plainview (NY): Cold Spring Harbor Lab Press; c1997.
· Ruegg MA; Bixby JL; (1998) Agrin orchestrates synaptic differentiation at the vertebrate neuromuscular junction. Trends Neuroscience 21, pp 22-27.
· Simpson J; *MG and Related Syndromes. Disorders of Voluntary Muscle* 5th ed., pp. 628-665,Walton Sir J; ed;Edinburgh, Churchill, Livingstone, 1988.
· Soliven B; Lang D; Penn A; et al; Seronegative MG: Neurology, 1988; 38: pp. 514-517.
· Stanley E; Drachman D; Stabilization of AChRs at Neuromuscular Junctions: Analysis by Specific Antibodies., *MG Biology and Treatment.* New York Academy of Sciences, Vol. 505, 1987. pp. 121-132.

## CHAPTER TWO:

· Aarli JA; Gilhus NE; Thorlacius S; et. al.; Recovery from global amnesia during plasma exchange in MG: report of a case. Acta Neurol Scand. 1989 Oct;80(4):351-3.
· Amino A; Shiozawa Z; Nagasaka T; et al; Sleep apnoea in well-controlled MG and the effect of thymectomy. J Neurol. 1998 Feb; 245 (2):77-80.
· Barthlen GM; Nocturnal respiratory failure as an indication of noninvasive ventilation in the patient with neuromuscular disease. Respiration 1997;64 Suppl 1:35-8.
· Gajdos P; Quera Salva MA; Respiratory disorders during sleep and myasthenia. Rev Neurol (Paris).2001 Nov;157(11 Pt 2):S145-7.
· Genkins G; Kornfeld P; Papatestas A;et al; Clinical Experience in More Than 2,000 Patients with MG. *MG Biology and Treatment.* New York Academy of Sciences, Vol. 505, 1987, pp. 500-516
· Iwasaki Y; Kinoshita M; Ikeda K; et. al.; Neuro-psychological function before and after plasma exchange in MG. J Neurol Sci.1993 Feb;114(2):223-6.
· Keesey JC; Does MG affect the brain? J Neurol Sci.1999 Nov 30;170 (2):77-89.
· Lang B; Vincent A; Autoantibodies to ion channels at the neuro-muscular junction. Autoimmun Rev.2003 Mar; 2(2):94-100.
· Lingwood-White F, ed; *The MG Companion* 2nd edition, British Association of Myasthenics and the MD Group of Great Britain, Jupiter Press Ltd., London, 1985, pp. 5-7.
· Manni R; Piccolo G; Sartori I; et al; Breathing during sleep in MG. Ital J Neurol Sci. 1995 Dec;16(9):589-94.

·   Mennuni G; Morante MT; Di Meo L; et al; Myasthenia and sleep. Schweiz Arch Neurol Neurochir Psychiatr.1983;133(2):193-203.
·   Newsom-Davies J; Willcox N; Schluep M; et al; Immunological Heterogeneity and Cellular Mechanisms in MG. *MG Biology and Treatment*. NY Acad of Sciences, Vol. 505, 1987, pp. 12-26.
·   Nicolle MW; Rask, S; Sleep Apnea in MG; Presentation; 2004 MGFA Scientific Meeting, Toronto. Neurology (in Press).
·   Nicolle MW; Personal Correspondence. 2 May, 2005.
·   Nicolle MW; MG. Neurolog. 2002 Jan;8(1):2-21.
·   Oger J; Research Update, Connections, MDA.12:1990 pp. 6-7.
·   Oosterhuis H; The Natural Course of MG; A Long Term Follow Up Study. Journal of Neurology, Neurosurgery and Psychiatry, 1989; 52: 1121-1127.
·   Quera-Salva MA; Guilleminault C; Chevret S; Troche G; Breathing disorders during sleep in MG. Ann Neurol.1992 Jan;31(1):86-92.
·   Simpson J; MG and Related Syndromes .*Disorders of Voluntary Muscle* 5[th]ed. pp. 628-665,Walton Sir J; ed;Edinburgh, Churchill, Livingstone, 1988.
·   Stepansky R; Zeitlhofer J; MG and sleep. Wien Klin Wochenschr.2001 Apr 17;113(7-8):285-7.
·   Stepansky R; Weber G; Zeitlhofer J; Sleep apnea and cognitive dysfunction in MG. Acta Med Austriaca.1997;24(3):128-31.
·   Stepansky R; Weber G; Zeitlhofer J; Sleep apnea in MG. Wien Med Wochenschr.1996;146(9-10):209-10.
·   Tucker D; Roeltgen D; Wann P; et al; Memory Dysfunction in MG:Evidence for Central Cholinergic Effects, Neurology, 1988; 38: pp. 1173-1177.

### CHAPTER THREE:

·   Barone D; Initial Evaluation Leading to the Diagnosis of MG. Summary of Oral Presentation Given to Garden State (N.J.) MG Foundation Chapter, May 1988.
·   Berrih-Aknin S; Morel E; Raimond F; et al.; The Role of the Thymus in MG. Immunohistological and Immunological Studies in 115 Cases. *MG Biology and Treatment*. NY Acad Sciences, Vol. 505, 1987, pp. 50-70.
·   Ellis FD; Hoyt CS; Ellis FJ; et. al.; Extra-ocular muscle responses to orbital cooling (ice test) for ocular MG diagnosis. JAAPOS.2000 Oct;4(5):271-81.
·   Ertas M; Arac N; Kumral K; Tuncbay T; Ice test as a simple diagnostic aid for MG. Acta Neurol Scand. 1994 Mar;89(3):227-9.

· Faure A; Gattegno L; Modigliani E; et al; Anti-bodies against myoid thymic cells and striated muscle, and monoclonal gammapathy in MG. Biomedicine.1975 Jun 30;23(6):241-5.
· Fujii Y; Monden Y. and Hashimoto J; AChR Antibody in MG:Sites of Production and Specific Activity. *MG Biology and Treatment.* NY Acad of Sciences, Vol. 505, 1987, pp.698-700.
· Golnik KC; Pena R; Lee AG; et.al.; An ice test for the diagnosis of MG. Ophthalmology. 1999 Jul;106(7):1282-6.
· Griffith H; *The Complete Guide to Medical Tests.* Fisher Books, Tucson, Arizona, 1988. pp.306-307.
· Hofstad H; Ulvestad E; Gilhus NE; et al; MG muscle antibodies examined by ELISA: IgG and IgM anti-bodies characterize different patient subgroups. Acta Neurol Scand.1992 Apr;85(4):233-8.
· Howard J.F. Jr; MG – A Summary; eMedicine.com, Inc. 2003,
· Ing EB; Ing SY; Ing T; Ramocki JA; The complication rate of edrophonium testing for suspected MG. Can J Ophthalmol.2000 Apr;35(3):141-4; 145.
· Koethe S; Du Pont B; Calvo A; et al.; Anti-AChR Antibodies in MG:Binding to Membrane-Bound Torpedo AChR. *MG Biology and Treatment.* NY Acadamy of Sciences, Vol. 505, 1987, pp. 557-565.
· Komiyama A; Hirayama K; Diagnostic usefulness of a hot test in patients with mild ocular MG. No To Shinkei.1987 Aug;39(8):733-7.
· Kubis KC; Danesh-Meyer HV; Savino PJ; et. al.; The ice test versus the rest test in MG.Ophthalmology. 2000 Nov;107(11):1995-8.
· Lertchavanakul A; Gamnerdsiri P; Hirunwiwatkul P; Ice test for ocular MG. J Med Assc Thai. 2001, Jun;84 Suppl.1:S131-6.
· Massey J;Sanders D and Howard J; The Effect of Cholinesterase Inhibitors on SFEMG in MG. Muscle and Nerve, 12: pp.154-155, 1989.
· Movaghar M; Slavin ML; Effect of local heat versus ice on blephar-optosis resulting from ocular myasthenia. Ophthalmology. 2000 Dec;107(12):2209-14.
· Mygland A; Tysnes OB; Aarli JA; et. al.; IgG subclass distribution of ryanodine receptor autoantibodies in patients with MG and thymoma. J Autoimmun. 1993 Aug;6(4):507-15.
· Nicolle MW; Personal Correspondence. 2 May, 2005.
· Nyberg-Hansen R and Gjerstad L; Immunopharmacological Treatment in MG: Transplantation Proceedings, Vol. XX, No. 3, Supl. 4, (June) 1988, pp. 201-210.
· Sanders D; The Electrodiagnosis of MG.*MG Biology and Treatment.* NY Academy of Sciences, Vol. 505, 1987, pp.539-556.

· Sethi KD; Rivner MH; Swift TR; Ice pack test for MG. Neurology.1987 Aug; 37(8):1383-5.
· Smith CI; Aarli JA; Hammarstrom L; Persson MA; IgG subclass distribution of MG thymoma-associated antiskeletal muscle antibodies. Neurology. 1984 Aug; 34(8):1094-6.
· Souan M; Geffard M; Vieillemaringe J; et al.; Anti-ACh Antibodies and the Pathogenesis of MG. *MG Biology and Treatment.* New York Academy of Sciences, Vol. 505, 1987, pp. 432-433

**CHAPTER FOUR:**
· Antozzi C; MG and myasthenic syndrome. Neurol Sci 2003 Oct;24 Suppl 4:S260-3.
· Berrih-Aknin, S; Morel, E; Raimond, F; et al.; The Role of the Thymus in MG. Immunohistological and Immunological Studies in 115 Cases. *MG Biology and Treatment*, Vol. 505, 1987, pp. 50-70.
· Besinger, U; Fateh-Moghadam, A; Knorr-Held, S; et al.; Immunomodulation in MG by High-Dose Intravenous 7-S Iggs. NY Acad of Sciences, Vol. 505, 1987, pp.828-831.
· Blossom GB; Ernstoff RM; Howells GA; et al; Thymectomy for MG. Arch Surg. 1993 Aug;128(8):855-62.
· Bonifati DM; Angelini C; Long-term cyclosporine treatment in a group of severe MG patients. J Neurol. 1997 Sep;244(9):542-7.
· Bramis J; Pikoulis E; Leppaniemi A; et al; Benefits of early thymectomy in patients with MG. Eur J Surg. 1997 Dec;163(12):897-902.
· Brenner T; Hamra-Amitay Y; Evron T; et al; The role of read through acetylcholinesterase in the pathophysiology of MG. FASEB J 2003 Feb;17(2):214-22
· Bril, V, Allenby K, Midroni G, et al. IGIV in neurology - evidence and recommendations. Can J Neurol Sci; 1999; Vol 26, 2; 139-152
· Caponnetto C; Rossi E; Primavera A; Mycophenolate mofetil: a new immunosuppressive approach. Successful treatment in a case of MG associated with incomplete lupus erythematosus syndrome and hepatitis C virus infection. Eur Neurol. 2001;46(1):53-4.
· Chaudhry V; Cornblath DR; Griffin JW; et al; Mycophenolate mofetil: a safe and promising immunosuppressant in neuromuscular diseases. Neurology. 2001 Jan 9; 56(1):94-96.
· Ciafaloni E; Massey JM; Tucker-Lipscomb et. al.; Mycophenolate mofetil for MG: an open-label pilot study. Neurology. 2001 Jan 9; 56 (1):97-99.
· Ciafaloni E; Nikhar NK; Massey JM; et. al.; Retrospective analysis of the use of cyclosporine in MG. Neurology. 2000 Aug 8;55(3):448-50.

· Callum JL and Pinkerton PH. *Bloody Easy; Blood transfusions, Blood Alternatives and Transfusion Reactions, A Guide to Transfusion Medicine.* Sunnybrook and Women's College Health Sciences Centre, 2003; ISBN 0-9681344-2-4.
· Canadian Pharmaceutical Assoc, Toronto, Canada. *Compendium of Pharmaceuticals and Specialties, 2004.*Refer to Product Monographs.
· Cornelio F; Peluchetti D; Mantegazza R; et al; The Course of MG in Patients Treated with Corticosteroids, Azathioprine and PE.*MG Biology and Treatment*, pp. 517-525.
· Dalakas MC; IV immune globulin therapy for neurologic diseases. Ann Intern Med.1997 May 1;126(9):721-30.
· de Oliveira JT; Campos GB; Cardoso FE; MG: results of thymectomy in 52 patients; Arq Neuropsiquiatr. 1995 Jun; 53(2):198-202.
· Evoli A; Batocchi A; Provenzano C; et al; Thymectomy in the Treatment of MG: Report of 247 Patients. J Neurol 1988.
· Fan Z; Wen G; Zhang Z; Thymectomy in the treatment of MG. Zhonghua Yi Xue Za Zhi. 1998 May;78(5):363-5.
· Gajdos P, Chevret S, Clair B, et al., for the Myasthenia Gravis Clinical Study Group. Clinical trial of plasma exchange and high-dose intravenous immunoglobulin in myasthenia gravis. Ann Neurol 1997;41: 789-796
· Gajdos, P; Outin, H; Morel, E; et al; High-Dose Intravenous Gg for MG: An alternative to PE? *MG Biology and Treatment,*pp. 842-844.
· Genkins, G; Kornfeld, P; Papatestas, A; et al; Clinical Experience in More Than 2,000 Patients with MG. *Ibid* pp. 500-516.
· Gerwitz, A; Molecular Medicine for Clinicians; The Prospects for Antisense Therapy. Hospital Practice: 1999:09.
· Goulon, M; Elkharrat, D; Lokiec, F; et al; Results of a One-Year Open Trial of CY-A in Ten Patients with Severe MG. Trans Proc, Vol. XX. No. 3, Suppl. 4 (June) 1988 pp. 211-217.
· Goulon, M; Elkharrat, D; Gajdos, P; et al; Preliminary Results in MG Treated with CY-A; *MG Biology and Treatment* pp. 857-860.
· Guillermo GR; Tellez-Zenteno JF; et al; Response of thymectomy: clinical and pathological characteristics among seronegative and seropositive MG patients. Acta Neurol Scand.2004 Mar;109(3):217-21.
· Grob, D; Arsur, E; Brunner, N; et al; The Course of MG and Therapies Affecting Outcome. *MG Biology and Treatment*, pp. 472-499
· Hauser RA; Malek AR; Rosen R; Successful treatment of a patient with severe refractory MG using mycophenolate mofetil. Neurol.1998 Sep; 51(3):912-3.

- Hatton, P; Diehl, J; Daly, B; et al; Transsternal Radical Thymectomy for MG:A 15-Year Review. The Annals of Thoracic Surgery, 47(6), June, 1090 pp. 838-840.
- Jaretzki A 3rd; Penn AS; Younger DS; et al; "Maximal" thymectomy for MG. Results. J Thorac Cardiovasc Surg.1988 May;95(5):747-57.
- Johns, T; Long-Term Corticosteroid Treatment of MG.*MG Biology and Treatment*, NY Acad of Sciences, pp. 568-583.
- Jongen JL, van Doorn PA, van der Meché FG, High-dose intravenous immunoglobulin therapy for myasthenia gravis. J Neurol 1998; 245; 26-31
- Kamolvarin N; Hemachudha T; Ongpipattanakul B; et al; Plasma C3c changes in MG patients receiving high-dose intravenous immuno-globulin during crisis. Acta Neurol Scand.1989 Oct;80(4):324-6.
- Kirmani JF; Yahia AM; Qureshi AI; Myasthenic Crisis. Curr Treat Options Neurol. 2004 Jan;6(1):3-15.
- Latov N; Chaudhry V; Koski CL; et al; Use of intravenous gamma globulins in neuroimmunologic diseases. J Allergy Clin Immunol. 2001 Oct;108(4 Suppl):S126-32.
- Louzir B; Ben Abdelhafidh N; Bahri M; et al; Association of systemic lupus erythematosis and MG. A new case report. Tunis Med.2003 Dec; 81(12):963-6.
- McKee, D; Agus, S; Soreq, H; et al; Antisense therapeutics in MG. Muscle disorders 2, 13th Meeting of the European Neurological Society, April 1, 2003.
- McEvoy, K; Windebank A; Daube J; Low P; 3,4-Diaminopyridine in the treatment of Lambert-Eaton myasthenic syndrome. *N. Engl. J. Med.* 321: 1567-1571, 1989.
- Maelicke, A; Yang, B; Sundaram, P; et al; Specific Immunosorbents in Diagnosis and Management of MG. *MG Biology and Treatment*, pp.669-675.
- Mantegazza, R; Antozzi C; Peluchetti, D; et al; Azathioprine as a Single Drug or in Combination with Steroids in the Treatment of MG.J Neurology (1980) 235: 449-453.
- Masaoka A; Yamakawa Y; et al; Extended thymectomy for MG patients: a 20-year review. Ann Thorac Surg.1996 Sep;62(3):853-9.
- Matell, G; Immunosuppressive Drugs: Azathioprine in the Treatment of MG. *MG Biology and Treatment*, pp. 588-594
- Melms, A; Endler, B; Kirchener, T; et al; The Thymus in MG: Functional and Morphological Studies. *Ibid* pp. 797-799.
- Meriggioli MN; Ciafaloni E; Al-Hayk KA; et al; Mycophenolate mofetil for MG: an analysis of efficacy, safety & tolerability; Neurol. 2003 Nov 25;61(10):1438-40.

· Meriggioli MN; Rowin J; Richman JG; et al; Mycophenolate mofetil for MG: a double-blind, placebo-controlled pilot study. Ann NY Acad Sci. 2003 Sep;998:494-9.

· Meriggioli MN; Treatment of MG with mycophenolate mofetil: a case report. Muscle Nerve.2000 Aug;23(8):1287-9.

· Miller, R; and Milner-Brown, H; Is There An Adverse Interaction between Corticosteroids and Anticholinesterase Drugs in Patients with MG? *MG Biology and Treatment* pp. 847-850.

· Molgo, J; Lemeignan,M; Lechat, P; Analysis of the action of 4-aminopyridine during repetitive stimulation at the neuromuscular junction. *Eur. J. Pharmacol.* 53: 307-311, 1979.

· Mowzoon N; Sussman A; Bradley WG; Mycophenolate (Cell-Cept) treatment of MG, chronic inflammatory polyneuropathy and inclusion body myositis. J Neurol Sci.2001 Apr 1;185(2):119-22.

· Newsom-Davis J; Therapy in MG and Lambert-Eaton myasthenic syndrome. Semin Neurol. 2003 Jun;23(2):191-8.

· Newsom-Davis, J; Willcox, N; Shluep, M; et al.; Immunological Heterogeneity and Cellular Mechanisms in MG. *MG Biology and Treatment*, pp. 12-26.

· Nicolle MW; Personal Correspondence. 2 May, 2005.

· Nyberg-Hansen, R and Gjerstad L; Immunopharmacological Treatment in MG: Transplantation Proceedings, Vol. XX, No. 3, Supl. 4, (June) 1988 pp. 201-210

· Oda, K; Ocular MG: Antibodies to End plates of Human Extraocular Muscle. *MG Biology and Treatment* pp. 861-863.

· Olanow, C; Wechsler, A; Sirotkin-Roses, M; et al; Thymectomy as Primary Therapy in MG. *Ibid.* pp. 595-606.

· Otto TJ; Strugalska H; Surgical treatment for MG. Thorax. 1987 Mar; 42(3):199-204.

· Papatestas, A; Kark, A; Bramis, J; et al; The Immediate Postoperative Complications and Long-Term Effects of Thymectomy in MG. *MG Biology and Treatment*, pp. 894-895.

· Richman DP; Agius MA; Treatment of autoimmune myasthenia gravis. Neurology. 2003 Dec 23;61(12):1652-61.

· Rowland, L; Chair of General Discussion on Therapy in MG. *MG Biology and Treatment*, pp. 607-609

· Sanders, DB; Personal Correspondence, 4th Oct.1991.

· Schalke, B; Kappos, L; Dommasch, D; et al; CY-A. Treatment of MG: Initial Results of a Double-Blind Trial of CY-A Versus Azathioprine. *MG Biology and Treatment*, pp.872-875.

· Schneider C; Gold R; Reiners K; Toyka KV; Mycophenolate mofetil in the therapy of severe MG. Eur Neurol.2001;46(2):79-82.

- Shorter, E; *The Health Century*, Doubleday, NY, pp. 32-37.
- Soreq H; Seidman S; Anti-sense approach to anticholinesterase therapeutics. Isr Med Assoc. J 2000 Jul;2 Suppl:81-5.
- Stangel M; Kiefer R; Pette M; et al; Side effects of intravenous immunoglobulins in neurological autoimmune disorders a prospective study. J Neurol. 2003 Jul;250(7):818-21.
- Thomsen, R; Wilson, D; Effects of 4-aminopyridine and 3,4-diaminopyridine on transmitter release at the neuromuscular junction. J. Pharmocol. Exp. Ther. 227: 260-265, 1983.
- Tindall, R; Rollins, J; Phillips, J; et al; A Double-Blind Randomized Placebo-Controlled Trial to Asses the Safety and Efficacy of CY-A in the Treatment of MG. *MG Biology and Treatment*, pp.854-856
- van Lunteren, E; Moyer, M; Electrophysiologic and Inotropic Effects of K+-Channel Blockade in Aged Diaphragm. Am J Respir Crit Care Med 158: 820-826 (1998).
- van Lunteren, E; Moyer, M; Effects of DAP on diaphragm force and fatigue, including fatigue due to neurotransmission failure. J. Appl. Physiol. 81(5): 2214-2220, 1996.
- Weder-Cisneros N; Tellez-Zenteno JF; et al; Response to thymectomy in patients with thymoma. Rev Invest Clin.2003 11-12;55(6):629-34.
- Wegner B, Ahmed I; Intravenous immunoglobulin monotherapy in long-term treatment of myasthenia gravis. Clin Neurol Neurosurg. 2002 Dec;105(1):3-8.
- Wittstock M; Benecke R; Zettl UK; Therapy with intravenous immunoglobulins: complications and side-effects. Eur Neurol. 2003;50(3):172-5.
- Younger, D; Jaretzki, A; Penn, A;et al; Maximum Thymectomy for MG. *MG Biology and Treatment*, pp. 832-835.
- Zweiman B; Theoretical mechanisms by which immuno-globulin therapy might benefit MG. Clin Immunol Immunopathol. 1989 Nov; 53(2 Pt 2):S83-91.

**CHAPTER FIVE:**

- Adelman HM; Winters PR; Mahan CS; et al; D-pen-induced MG: diagnosis obscured by coexisting chronic obstructive pulmonary disease. Am J Med Sci. 1995 Apr;309(4):191-3.
- Andonopoulos AP; Terzis E; Tsibri E; et al; D-penicillamine induced MG in rheumatoid arthritis: an unpredictable common occurrence? Clin Rheumatol.1994 Dec;13(4):586-8.
- Childs L; Harrison R; and Lunt G; Complement-Mediated Muscle Damage Produced by Myasthenic Sera. *MG Biology and Treatment.*, NY Academy of Sciences, Vol. 505, 1987. pp. 180-193.

· Drachman D; De Silva S; Ramsay D; et al; Humoral Pathogenesis of MG.*MG Biology and Treatment.* pp. 90-105.
· Drosos AA; Christou L; Galanopoulou V; et al; D-pen induced MG: clinical, serological and genetic findings. Clin Exp Rheumatol.1993 Jul-Aug;11(4):387-91.
· Dwyer D; Vakil M; Bradley R; et al; A Possible Cause of MG: Idiotypic Networks Involving Bacterial Antigens. ibid. pp. 461-471.
· Euler HH; Marmont AM; Bacigalupo A; et al; Early recurrence or persistence of autoimmune diseases after unmanipulated autologous stem-cell transplantation. Blood. 1996 Nov 1; 88(9):3621-5.
· Evoli A; Batocchi AP; Minisci C; et al; Therapeutic options in ocular MG. Neuromuscul Disord. 2001 Mar;11(2):208-16.
· Evoli A; Tonali PA; Padua L; et. al; Clinical correlates with anti-MuSK antibodies in generalized seronegative MG. Brain 2003 Oct;126(Pt 10):2304-11.
· Gronseth GS,    Barohn RJ; Thymectomy for Myasthenia Gravis. Current Treatment Options in Neurology 2002, 4:203-209
· Gutmann L; Phillips LH 2nd; Gutmann L; Trends in the association of Lambert-Eaton myasthenic syndrome with carcinoma. Neurology. 1992 Apr;42(4):848-50.
· Hoch W; McConville J; Helms S; et. al; Auto-antibodies to the receptor tyrosine kinase MuSK in patients with MG without AChR antibodies. Nature Med, 7; 365-368. (2001).
· Ikehara S; Bone marrow transplantation: a new strategy for intractable diseases. Drugs Today (Barc). 2002 Feb;38(2):103-11.
· Ikehara S; Bone marrow transplantation for autoimmune diseases. Acta Haematol. 1998; 99(3):116-32.
· Jaretzki et al.; Myasthenia gravis: Recommendations for clinical research standards. *Neurology.*2000; 55: 16-23.
· Kato Y; Naito Y; Narita Y; et.al.; D-penicillamine-induced MG in a case of eosinophilic fasciitis. Neurol Sci. 1997 Feb 27; 146(1):85-6.
· Kupersmith MJ; Latkany R; Homel P; Development of generalized disease at two years in patients with ocular MG. Arch Neurol.2003 Feb; 60(2): 243-8.
· Kupersmith MJ; Moster M; Bhuiyan S; et al; Beneficial effects of corticosteroids on ocular MG. Arch Neurol.1996 Aug;53(8):802-4.
· Lefvert A; Holm G; Pirskanen R; Autoantiidiotypic Antibodies in MG. *MG Biology and Treatment.* pp.133.154.
· Lang B; Vincent A; Autoantibodies to ion channels at the NMJ. Autoimmun Rev. 2003 Mar; 2(2):94-100.

· Lennon VA; Kryzer TJ; Griesman GE; et al; Calcium-Channel Antibodies in the Lambert-Eaton Syndrome and other Para-neoplastic Syndromes. New Eng Jour Med Vol 332: 1467 June 1, 1995, no 22.

· Maddison P; Newsom-Davis J;Treatment for LEMS. Cochrane Database Syst Rev. 2003;(2):CD003279.

· Mee J; Paine M; Byrne E; et al; Immunotherapy of ocular MG reduces conversion to generalized MG. J. Neuro-ophthalmol.2003 Dec;23(4): 251-5.

· Monsul NT; Patwa HS; Knorr AM; et al; The effect of prednisone on the progression from ocular to generalized MG. J Neurol Sci.2004 Feb 15;217(2):131-3.

· Megeath LJ; Kirber MT; Hopf C; et al; Calcium-dependent maintenance of agrin-induced postsynaptic specializations. Neuroscience. 2003;122(3):659-68.

· Nakamura H; Taniguchi Y; Suzuki Y; et al; Delayed remission after thymectomy for MG of the purely ocular type J Thorac Cardiovasc Surg.1996 Aug;112(2):371-5.

· Newsom-Davis J; Lambert-Eaton myasthenic syndrome. Rev Neurol (Paris).2004 Feb;160(2):177-80.

· Newsom-Davis J; Therapy in MG and LEMS. Semin Neurol. 2003 Jun; 23(2):191-8.

· Nicolle MW; Personal Correspondence, 2 May 2005.

· Nicolle MW; MG. Neurolog. 2002 Jan;8(1):2-21.

· Oda, K; Ocular MG: Antibodies to End plates of Human Extraocular Muscle. *MG Biology and Treatment.* pp. 861-863.

· Oosterhuis H; The Natural Course of MG; A Long Term Follow Up Study. Journal of Neurology, Neurosurgery and Psychiatry, 1989; 52: 1121-1127.

· Pestronk A; Drachman D; Antibody-Mediated Membrane Abnormalities in PM: Reduction of AChRs by Igg. *MG Biology and Treatment.* NY Acad of Sciences, Vol. 505, 1987 pp. 357-367.

· Plested CP; Tang T; Spreadbury I; AChR phosphorylation and indirect inhibition of AChR function in seronegative MG. Neurology.2002 Dec 10;59(11):1682-8.

· Ramsay DA; Drachman DB; Drachman RJ; et al; Stabilization of acetylcholine receptors at the neuromuscular synapse: the role of the nerve. Brain Res. 1992 May 29;581(2):198-207.

· Roberts PF; Venuta F; Rendina E; et al; Thymectomy in the treatment of ocular MG. J Thorac Cardiovasc Surg. 2001 Sep;122(3):562-8.

· Soliven B.; Lang D; Penn A; et al.; Seronegative MG: Neurology, 1988; 38: pp. 514-517.

- Sommer N; Sigg B; Melms A; et al; Ocular MG: response to long-term immunosuppressive treatment. J Neurol Neurosurg Psychiatry.1997 Feb;62(2):156-62.
- Stanley E; Drachman D.; Stabilization of AChRs at Neuromuscular Junctions: Analysis by Specific Antibodies. *MG Biology and Treatment.* pp. 121-132.
- Stefansson K; Dieperink M; Richman D; et al; Sharing of Epitopes by Bacteria and the Nicotinic AChR: A Possible Role in the Pathogenesis of MG. *MG Biology and Treatment.* pp.451-460.
- Thomas CR, Wright CD, Loehrer PJ. *Thymoma: state of the art.* J Clin Oncol 1999;17:2280-9.
- Vincent A; Bowen J; Newsom-Davis J; et al; Seronegative generalised MG: clinical features, antibodies, and their targets. Lancet Neurol. 2003 Feb; 2(2):99-106.
- Wirtz PW; Sotodeh M; Nijnuis M; et al; Difference in distribution of muscle weakness between MG and the Lambert-Eaton myasthenic syndrome. J Neurol Neurosurg Psychiatry. 2002 Dec;73(6): 766-8.
- Yang DS; Nakahara K; Ohno K; et al; The result of extended thymectomy in patients with MG of pure ocular type. Nippon Kyobu Geka Gakkai Zasshi.1989 Feb; 37(2):313-7.

**CHAPTER SIX:**
- Bady B; Chauplannaz G; Carrier H; Congenital Lambert-Eaton myasthenic syndrome. J Neurol Neurosurg Psychiatry.1987 Apr;50(4): 476-8.
- Banwell BL, Ohno K, Sieb JP, Engel AG.; Novel truncating RAPSN mutations causing congenital myasthenic syndrome responsive to 3,4-diaminopyridine. Neuromuscul Disord. 2004 Mar;14(3):202-7.
- Becker, W; *The World of the Cell.* eds, Behnke, JW; Gillen, JR; 1986 Benjamin/Cummings Pub. Co. Menlo Park CA.
- Beeson D; Brydson M; Betty M; et al; Primary structure of the human muscle AChR. cDNA cloning of the gamma and epsilon subunits. Eur J Biochem. 1993 Jul 15;215(2):229-38.
- Brehm, P, Ono F, Shcherbatko A, et al; The Zebra fish Motility Mutant *twitch once* Reveals New Roles for Rapsyn in Synaptic Function; J Neurosi, Aug 1, 2002, 22(15):6491-6498
- Brownlow S; Webster R; Croxen R; et al; AChR delta subunit mutations underlie a fast-channel myasthenic syndrome and arthrogryposis multiplex congenita. J Clin Invest. 2001 Jul;108(1): 125-30.

·   Burke G; Cossins J; Maxwell S; Owens G; et al; Rapsyn mutations in hereditary myasthenia: Distinct early- and late-onset phenotypes. Neurol. 2003 Sep 23;61(6):826-828.
·   Chevessier F, Faraut B, Ravel-Chapuis A, Richard P, Gaudon K, et al.; MUSK, a new target for mutations causing congenital myasthenic syndrome. Hum Mol Genet. 2004 Dec 15;13(24):3229-40.
·   Croxen R; Vincent A; Newsom-Davis J; et. al.; MG in a woman with congenital AChR deficiency due to epsilon-subunit mutations. Neurol. 2002 May 28; 58(10):1563-5.
·   Croxen R; Hatton C; Shelley C; et al; Recessive inheritance and variable penetrance of slow-channel congenital myasthenic syndrome. Neurol. 2002 Jul 23;59(2):162-8.
·   Croxen R; Newland C; Beeson D; et al; Mutations in different functional domains of the human muscle AChR alpha subunit in patients with the slow-channel Congenital Myasthenic Syndrome. Hum Mol Genet.1997 May; 6(5):767-74.
·   Donger C; Krejci E; Serradell AP; et al; Mutation in the human AChsE -associated collagen gene, COLQ, is responsible for congenital myasthenic syndrome with endplate AChsE deficiency (Type Ic). (1998) Am. J. Hum. Genet. 63:967-975
·   Dunne V; Maselli RA; Identification of pathogenic mutations in the human rapsyn gene. J Hum Genet.2003;48(4):204-7.
·   Engel AG; Uchitel OD; Walls TJ; et al; Newly recognized congenital myasthenic syndrome associated with high conductance and fast closure of the AChR channel. Ann Neurol. 1993 Jul;34(1):38-47.
·   Engel AG; Ohno K; Sine SM; Congenital Myasthenic Syndrome: progress over the past decade. Muscle Nerve.2003 Jan;27(1):4-25.
·   Engel AG; Ohno K; Shen XM; et.al.; Congenital Myasthenic Syndrome: multiple molecular targets at the neuromuscular junction. NY Acad Sci. 2003 Sep;998:138-60.
·   Furui E; Fukushima K; et al; Familial limb girdle myasthenia with tubular aggregates. Muscle Nerve.1997 May;20(5):599-603.
·   Fukudome T; Ohno K; Brengman JM; Engel AG; Quinidine normalizes the open duration of slow-channel mutants of the AChR. Neuroreport. 1998 Jun 1;9(8):1907-11.
·   García-Colunga J; Awad JN; Miled R; Blockage of muscle and neuronal nAChRs by fluoxetine (Prozac). Proc. Natl. Acad. Sci. USA Vol. 94, pp. 2041-2044, March 1997 Pharmacol.
·   Goldhammer Y; Blatt I; Sadeh M; et. al.; Congenital myasthenia associated with facial malformations in Iraqi and Iranian Jews. A new genetic syndrome. Brain.1990 Oct;113 ( Pt 5):1291-306.

- Gomez CM; Maselli RA; Groshong J; et al; Active calcium accumulation underlies severe weakness in a panel of mice with slow-channel syndrome. J Neurosci. 2002 Aug 1;22(15):6447-57.
- Grosman C; Salamone FN; Sine SM; et. al.; The extracellular linker of muscle AChR channels is a gating control element. Gen Physiol. 2000 Sep;116(3):327-40.
- Harper CM; Congenital myasthenic syndromes.Semin Neurol. 2004 Mar;24(1):111-23.
- Harper C; Fukodome T; Engel A; Treatment of slow-channel congenital myasthenic syndrome with fluoxetine. Neurol. 2003 May 27;60(10)1710-3.
- Harper CM; Engel AG; Quinidine sulfate therapy for the slow-channel congenital myasthenic syndrome. Ann Neurol. 1998 Apr;43(4):480-4.
- Hatton CJ; Shelley C; Brydson M; et al; Properties of the human muscle nicotinic receptor, and of the slow-channel congenital myasthenic syndrome mutant epsilon-L221F, inferred from maximum likelihood fits. J Physiol. 2003 Mar 15;547(Pt 3):729-60.
- Hutchinson DO; Walls TJ; Nakano S; et al; Congenital end-plate acetylcholinesterase deficiency. Brain. 1993 Jun;116 ( Pt 3):633-53.
- Martinou J; Falls DL; Fischbach GD; Ach-Inducing Activity Stimulates Expression of the e-Subunit Gene of the Muscle AChR. Proc Nat Acad of Sci, Vol 88, pp 7669-7673.
- Maselli RA; Kong DZ; Bowe CM; et al; Presynaptic CMS due to quantal release deficiency. Neurology.2001 Jul 24;57(2):279-89.
- Menold MM; Sadeh M; Lennon F; et al; Evidence for genetic heterogeneity supports clinical differences in congenital myasthenic syndrome. Hum Hered.1998 Nov-Dec;48(6):325-32.
- Muller JS; Mildner G; Muller-Felber; et al; Rapsyn N88K is a frequent cause of congenital myasthenic syndrome in European patients. Neurology.2003 Jun 10;60(11):1805-10.
- Nicolle MW; Personal Correspondence. 2 May, 2005.
- Ohno K; Quiram PA; Milone M; et al; CMS due to heteroallelic nonsense/missense mutations in the AChR epsilon sub-unit gene: identification and functional characterization of six new mutations. Hum Mol Genet. 1997 May;6(5):753-66.
- Ohno K; Engel AG; Shen XM; Selcen D; et al; Rapsyn mutations in humans cause endplate AChR deficiency and myasthenic syndrome. Am J Hum Genet. 2002 Apr;70(4):875-85.
- Ohno K; Tsujino A; Brengman JM; et al; Choline acetyltransferase mutations cause myasthenic syndrome associated with episodic apnea in humans. Proc Natl Acad Sci2001 Feb 13;98(4):2017-22.

- Ohno K; Engel AG; Brengman JM; et al; The spectrum of mutations causing end-plate ACh deficiency.(2000) Ann. Neurol. 47:162-170.
- Ohno K; Brengman J; Tsujino A; Human endplate ACh deficiency caused by mutations in the collagen-like tail subunit (ColQ) of the asymmetric enzyme. Proc Natl Acad Sci 1998 Aug 4;95(16):9654-9.
- Ohno, K; Wang, H.L; Milone M; et al; Congenital myasthenic syndrome caused by decreased agonist binding affinity due to a mutation in the AChR [epsilon] subunit. Neuron, 17, 157-170 (1996).
- Rodolico C; Toscano A; Autunno M; et al; Limb-girdle myasthenia: clinical, electrophysiological and morphological features in familial and autoimmune cases. Neuromuscul Disord.2002 Dec;12(10):964-9.
- Sadeh M; Blatt I; Goldhammer Y; Single fiber EMG in a congenital myasthenic syndrome associated with facial malformations. Muscle Nerve.1993 Feb;16(2):177-80.
- Shankar A; Solomon T; Joseph TP; et al; Autosomal recessive limb girdle myasthenia in two sisters. Neurol India. 2002 Dec;50(4):500-3.
- Shapira YA; Sadeh ME; Bergtraum MP; et al; Three novel COLQ mutations and variation of phenotypic expressivity due to G240X. Neurol. 2002 Feb 26;58(4):603-9.
- Shen XM; Ohno K; Fukudome T; et al; CMS caused by low-expressor fast-channel AChR delta subunit mutation. Neurology. 2002 Dec 24;59(12):1881-8.
- Sieb JP; Tolksdorf K; Dengler R; et al; An autosomal-recessive CMS with tubular aggregates in a Libyan family. Neuromuscul Disord.1996 Mar;6(2):115-9.
- Sine SM; Wang HL; Ohno K; et al; Mechanistic diversity underlying fast channel congenital myasthenic syndromes. Ann N Y Acad Sci. 2003 Sep; 998:128-37.
- Sine SM; Ohno K; Bouzat C; et al; Mutation of the AChR alpha subunit causes a slow-channel myasthenic syndrome by enhancing agonist binding affinity. Neuron.1995 Jul;15(1):229-39.
- Tsujino A; Maertens C; Ohno K; et al; Myasthenic syndrome caused by mutation of the SCN4A sodium channel. Proc Natl Acad Sci 2003 Jun 10;100(12):7377-82.

- Witzemann V; Schwarz H; Koenen M; et al; AChR epsilon-subunit deletion causes muscle weakness and atrophy in juvenile and adult mice; Proc. Natl. Acad. Sci. Vol. 93, pp. 13286-13291, November 1996;
- Zammarchi E; Donati MA; Masi S; et al; Familial infantile myasthenia: a neuromuscular cause of respiratory failure. Childs Nerv Syst.1994 Jul;10(5):347-9.

**CHAPTER SEVEN:**

· Afifi AK; Bell WE.; Tests for juvenile MG: comparative diagnostic yield and prediction of outcome. Child Neurol. 1993 Oct;8(4):403-11.

· Ahlsten G; Lefvert AK; Osterman PO; et al; Follow-up study of muscle function in children of mothers with MG during pregnancy. J Child Neurol. 1992 Jul;7(3):264-9.

· Anlar B; Ozdirim E; Renda Y; et al; MG in childhood. Acta Paediatr. 1996 Jul;85(7):838-42.

· Batocchi AP, Majolini L, Evoli A, et. al.: Course and treatment of myasthenia gravis during pregnancy. Neurology 1999, 52(3):447-52.

· Batocchi AP; Evoli A; Palmisani MT; et al; Early-onset MG: clinical characteristics and response to therapy. Eur J Pediatr.1990 Nov;150 (1):66-8.

· Bergoffen J; Zmijewski CM; Fischbeck KH; Familial autoimmune MG. Neurology.1994 Mar;44(3 Pt 1):551-4.

· Burke ME; MG and pregnancy. J Perinat Neonatal Nurs. 1993, Jun;7 (1):11-21.

· DeWitte DB; Buick MK; Cyran SE; et. al.; Neonatal pancytopenia and severe combined immunodeficiency associated with ante-natal administration of azathioprine and prednisone. J Pediatr.1984 Oct;105 (4):625-8.

· Eden R; Gall A; MG and Pregnancy. A Reappraisal of Thymectomy. Obstetrics and Gynecology 62:328, 1983

· Engel AG; Ohno K; Sine SM; Congenital myasthenic syndromes: progress over the past decade. Muscle Nerve.2003 Jan;27(1):4-25.

· Essa M; El-Medany Y; Hajjar W; et al; Maximal thymectomy in children with MG. Eur J Cardiothorac Surg. 2003 Aug;24(2):187-91.

· Evoli A; Batocchi AP; Bartoccioni E; et al; Juvenile MG with prepubertal onset. Neuromuscul Disord.1998 Dec;8(8):561-7.

· Evoli A; Batocchi AP; et al; Familial autoimmune MG: report of four families. J Neurol Neurosurg Psych.1995 Jun;58(6):729-31.

· Fennell D; Ringel S; MG and Pregnancy. Obstetrical and Gynecological Survey, 1987, Vol. 4, No. 7. pp. 414-419.

· Fraser D;Turner J; MG and Pregnancy Proc. Royal Society of Medicine 56:379, 1983.

· Garofalo-Gomez N; Sardinas-Hernandez NL; et al; MG in infancy. A report of 12 cases; Rev Neurol. 2002 May 16-31;34(10):908-11.

· Giwa-Osagie O; Newton J; Archer V; Obstetrical Performance of Patients with MG. Int. Journal Gynecology and Obstetrics 19:267, 1981.

· Hoff JM; Daltveit AK; Gilhus NE; MG: Consequences for pregnancy, delivery, and the newborn. Neurology. 2003 Nov 25;61(10):1362-6.

- Honeybourne D; Dyer PA; Mohr PD; Familial MG. J Neurol Neurosurg Psychiatry.1982 Sep;45(9):854-6.
- Licht C; Model P; Kribs A; et al; Transient neonatal MG. Nervenarzt. 2002 Aug;73(8):774-8.
- Mitchell PJ, Bebbington M: Myasthenia gravis in pregnancy. Obstet Gynecol 1992, 80(2):178-81. 7.
- Norgard B; Pedersen L; Fonager K; et al; Azathioprine, mercaptopurine and birth outcome: a population-based cohort study. Aliment Pharmacol Ther.2003 Mar 15;17(6):827-34.
- Nicolle MW; Personal Correspondence. 2 May, 2005.
- Nicolle MW; Koopman, W. MG and Pregnancy. Patient Handout. April 2005.
- Picone O; Audibert F; Gajdos P; et al; MG and pregnancy: report on 13 cases. J Gynecol Obstet Biol Reprod. 2003 Nov;32(7):654-9.
- Raksadawan N; Kankirawatana P; Balankura K;et al; Childhood onset MG. J Med Assoc Thai. 2002 Aug;85 Suppl 2: S769-77.
- Schrecter J; Poliovirus Vaccine and Child Care. The Link March - April, 1991.
- Sieb JP; Kraner S; Steinlein OK; Congenital myasthenic syndromes. Semin Pediatr Neurol. 2002 Jun;9(2):108-119.
- Skelly CL; Jackson CC; Wu Y; et al; Thoracoscopic thymectomy in children with MG. Am Surg. 2003 Dec; 69(12):1087-1089.
- Tallent MB; Simmons RL; Najarian JS; Birth defects in child of male recipient of kidney transplant. JAMA.1970 Mar 16;211(11):1854-5.
- Tan JH; Ho KH; Familial autoimmune MG. Singapore Med J. 2001 Apr;42(4):178-9.
- Téllez-Zenteno JF, Hernández-Ronquillo L, Vicente Salinas B, Orlandoda Silva E: Myasthenia gravis and pregnancy: clinical implications and neonatal outcome  BMC Musculoskeletal Disorders 2004, 5:42
- Williamson RA; Karp LE; Azathioprine teratogenicity: review of the literature and case report. Obstet Gynecol.1981 Aug;58(2):247-50.
- Zlatanic J; Korelitz BI; Rajapakse R; et al; Complications of pregnancy and child development after cessation of treatment with 6-mercaptopurine for inflammatory bowel disease. J Clin Gastroenterol.2003 Apr;36(4):303-9.

**CHAPTER EIGHT:**

- Aggarwal A; Gupta D; Behera D; et al; Intensive respiratory care in patients with myasthenic crisis. Neurol India 2002; 50:348-51.
- Bedlack R; Sanders D; How to handle myasthenic crisis. Essential steps in patient care. Postgrad Med. 2000 Apr;107(4):211-4, 220-2.

· Liverani, L; Cold Turkey, RN Magazine quoted by MG Assoc., Portland, Oregon, undated.
· Maelicke, A; Yang,B; Sundaram, P; et al; Specific Immunosorbents in Diagnosis and Management of MG, *MG Biology and Treatment,* NY Academy of Sciences, Vol 505, 1987 pp.669-675.
· Miller, R; Recent Advances in the Treatment of MG: *Contact*, Newsletter of the MG, Toronto Chapter of the MDA, Undated pp. 13-14.
· MG Foundation Inc. *MG:The Disease, A Case History* pp. 12.
· Nicolle MW; Personal Correspondence. 2 May, 2005.
· The MG Foundation Inc. The; *MG:A Manual for the Physician*, Oct., 1985. pp. 16-18
· Rhynsburger, J; MG Survival Guide: A Guide to Patient-Directed Health Management (MG Foundation Inc.)

**CHAPTER NINE:**

· Benson, H; Stark, M; *Timeless Healing: The Power and Biology of Belief*, Scribner, 1996.
· Hackett, T; Cassen, N; eds, *Massachusetts General Hospital Handbook of General Hospital Psychiatry.*
· Kubler-Ross E; *On Death and Dying*, Macmillan, NY, 1969.
· Lewis, K; Grief in Chronic Illness and Disability. Journal of Rehabilitation, July-Sept., 1983
· Nicolle MW; Personal Correspondence. 2 May, 2005.
· Ornish, D; *Love & Survival: The Scientific Basis for the Healing Power of Intimacy*, Harper Collins, 1998.
· Scott, David; *Easy-to-Use Zen*, Vega Pub. London, 2002.
· Werner-Beland, J; ed. Physical Disability and Grief Resolution; pp 47-61, *Grief Responses to Long-Term Illness and Disability;* Reston Pub, 1980.

**CHAPTER TEN:**

· Argov Z; Brenner T; Abramsky O; Ampicillin may aggravate clinical and experimental MG. Arch Neurol.1986 Mar;43(3):255-6.
· Boneva N; Brenner T; Argov Z; Gabapentin may be hazardous in MG. Muscle Nerve. 2000 Aug;23(8):1204-8.
· Booker HE; Chun RW; Sanguino M; MG syndrome associated with trimethadione. JAMA.1970; Jun 29;212(13):2262-3.
· Booker HE; Chun RW; Sanguino M; Myasthenic syndrome associated with trimethadione. Neurology. 1968 Mar;18(3):274.
· Brumlik J; Jacobs RS; MG associated with diphenylhydantoin therapy for epilepsy. J Pharm Pharmacol. 1987 Nov;39(11):896-9.

· Cadisch R; Streit E; Hartmann K; Exacerbation of pseudo-paralytic MG following azithromycin (Zithromax) Schweiz Med Wochenschr.1996 Feb 24;126(8):308-10.

· David, N; Muscle-Relaxing Drugs MG Patients Should Avoid, (list) University of Oregon Medical School, Pharmacology Dept.

· Drachman DA; Skom JH; Procainamide---a hazard in MG. Arch Neurol.1965 Sep;13(3):316-20.

· Fiekers JF; Sites and mechanisms of antibiotic-induced neuromuscular block: a pharmacological analysis using quantal content, voltage clamped end-plate currents and single channel analysis. Acta Physiol Pharmacol Ther Latinoam. 1999;49(4):242-50.

· García-Colunga J; Awad JN; Miled R; Blockage of muscle and neuronal nicotinic acetylcholine receptors by fluoxetine(Prozac). *Proc. Natl. Acad. Sci. USA Vol. 94*, pp. 2041-2044, March 1997 Pharmacol.

· Gilbert GJ; MG and epilepsy. J Fla Med Assoc.1970 May;57(5):34-5.

· Godley PJ; Morton TA; Karboski JA; Tami JA; Procainamide-induced myasthenic crisis. Ther Drug Monit. 1990 Jul;12(4):411-4.

· Gurtubay IG; Morales G; Arechaga O; et al; Development of MG after interferon alpha therapy. Electromyogr Clin Neurophysiol.1999 Mar;39(2):75-8.

· Harada H; Tamaoka A; Kohno Y; et al; Exacerbation of MG in a patient after interferon-beta treatment for chronic active hepatitis C. J Neurol Sci.1999 Jun 1;165(2):182-3.

· Johnson Williams N; Schuman, N; The curved-bristle toothbrush: an aid for the handicapped population. J of Dentistry For Children, July-August 1988.

· Jonkers I; Swerup C; Pirskanen R; et al; Acute effects of intravenous injection of beta-adrenoreceptor- and calcium channel at antagonists and agonists in MG. Muscle Nerve.1996 Aug;19(8):959-65.

· Kaeser HE; Drug-induced myasthenic syndromes. Acta Neurol Scand Suppl.1984;100:39-47.

· Khella SL; Kozart D; Unmasking and exacerbation of MG by ophthalmic solutions: betoxolol, tobramycin, and dexamethasone. A case report. Muscle Nerve.1997 May;20(5):631.

· Komar J; Szalay M; Szel I; A myasthenic episode following intake of large amounts of a beta blocker. Fortschr Neurol Psychiatr.1987 Jun;55(6):201-2.

· Krendel DA; Hopkins LC; Adverse effect of verapamil in a patient with LEMS. Muscle Nerve.1986 Jul-Aug; 9(6):519-22.

- Lee DC; Kim YI; Liu HH; Johns TR; Presynaptic and postsynaptic actions of procainamide on neuromuscular transmission. Muscle Nerve.1983 Jul-Aug;6(6):442-7.
- Lee SC; Ho ST; Acute effects of verapamil on neuromuscular transmission in patients with MG. Proc Natl Sci Counc Repub China B.1987 Jul;11(3):307-12.
- May EF; Calvert PC; Aggravation of MG by erythromycin. Ann Neurol. 1990 Oct;28(4):577-9.
- Meriney SD; Hulsizer SC; Lennon VA; et. al.;; Lambert-Eaton myasthenic syndrome immunoglobulins react with multiple types of calcium channels in small-cell lung carcinoma. Ann Neurol.1996 Nov;40(5):739-49.
- Nicolle MW; Personal Correspondence. 2 May, 2005.
- The MG Foundation, Inc. The. Greater Chicago Area Chapter. *Patient to Patient Memo:A Handbook of Hints for MG Patients.*
- The MG Foundation Inc., *MG:A Manual for the Physician*, Oct., 1985. pp. 15-16.
- The MG Foundation Inc., *MG:A Manual for the Nurse*, pp. 12, 18-19 1985.
- Osserman KE; Genkins G; Studies in MG: review of a 20 year experience in over 1200 patients. Mt. Sinai Journal of Medicine 1971;38:497-572.
- Ozawa T; Nakajima T; Furui E; et.al; A case of MG associated with long-term phenytoin therapy.Rinsho Shinkeigaku.1996 Nov;36(11): 1262-4.
- Peterson H; Association of trimethadione therapy and MG. N Engl J Med. 1966 Mar 3;274(9):506-7.
- Pina Latorre MA; Cobeta JC; Rodilla F; et al; Influence of calcium antagonist drugs in MG in the elderly. J Clin Pharm Ther.1998 Oct;23 (5):399-401.
- Protti DA; Reisin R; Mackinley TA; Uchitel OD; Calcium channel blockers & transmitter release at the normal human neuromuscular junction. Neurol 1996;46:1391-1396.
- Rotenberg, G; ed. *Compendium of Pharmaceuticals and Specialties,* Canadian Pharmaceutical Assoc., Toronto, Ont.
- Scheschonka A; Beuche W; Treatment of post-herpetic pain in MG: exacerbation of weakness due to gabapentin. Pain.2003 Jul;104(1-2): 423-4.
- Singh YN; Marshall IG; et. al. Reversal of antibiotic-induced muscle weakness by 3,4-DAP J Pharm Pharmacol.1978 Apr;30(4):249-50.
- Stoffer SS; Chandler JH; Quinidine-induced exacerbation of MG in patient with Graves' disease. Arch Intern Med.1980 Feb;140(2):283-4.

· Swash M; Ingram DA; Adverse effect of verapamil in MG. Muscle Nerve.1992 Mar;15(3):396-8.
· Zhi-Qiang, C; FMG: Report of 7 Cases in 3 Families. Chinese Medical Journal, 99(9): pp. 749-750, 1986

**CHAPTER ELEVEN:**
· Heruti RJ; Levy A; Adunski A; Conversion motor paralysis disorder: overview and rehab model. Spinal Cord.2002 Jul;40(7):327-34.
· Knieling J; Weiss H; Faller H; et al; Follow-up of MG. Results of a longitudinal study of the significance of psycho-social predictors. Nervenarzt.1998 Feb;69(2):137-44.
· Nicholson, G; Wilby, J; Tennant, C; MG:The Problem of a 'Psychiatric' Misdiagnosis. The Medical Journal of Australia, June 9, 1986, Vol. 144 pp.632-638.
· Nicolle MW; Personal Correspondence. 2 May, 2005.
· Rohr, W; MG in the frontier of psychiatric diagnosis. Psychiatr Prax.1992 Sep;19(5):157-63.
· Santy, P; Undiagnosed MG in Emergency Psychiatric Referrals. Annals of Emer Med, 12:6, June, 1983 pp. 397-398.
· Sheddon, J; MG:A Study of Social, Medical and Emotional Problems in 26 Patients:The Lancet, March 8, 1980 pp. 526-528.
· Tennant, C; Wilby, J; Nicholson, G; Psychological Correlates ofMG:A Brief Report.Journal of Psychosomatic Research, Vol. 30, No. 5, pp. 575-580, 1986.
· Vellodi, C; and Tallis, R; Unusual Case of MG in an Elderly Patient with Severe Muscular Atrophy; Gerontology 34: 209-211 (1988).

**APPENDIX:**
· Criteria for Somatization Disorder summarized from: American Psychiatric Association. (1994). *Diagnostic and statistical manual of mental disorders, fourth edition.* Washington, DC: Amer Psych Assc

# Biographies

## Deborah Cavel-Greant

Deborah's career as a journalist began during her teens. Over the years she worked on-staff at newspapers, magazines and at the Museum of Northern British Columbia, where she co-authored a textbook on the natural history of the Canadian Pacific Northcoast. An interest in health care led her to focus her writing in that area in the early 70s. In the late 1970s she became a Certified Herbalist. She is currently pursuing her Master Herbalist designation.

While it was initially believed that Deborah had MG, further diagnostic study proved that she has, not MG, but the inherited ion channel disorder Hypokalemic Periodic Paralysis.

## Michael W. Nicolle, MD, FRCPC, D.Phil.

Dr. Nicolle completed medical school at the University of Western Ontario in London, Ontario, Canada in 1985 and finished his residency training in neurology in 1990. His interest in myasthenia gravis started with a patient encounter in the middle of his neurology residency, which led to further Fellowship Training at the University of Oxford (England) between 1991 and 1994. At Oxford, Dr. Nicolle was involved in research projects looking at the development of more specific immunotherapies in myasthenia gravis.

As staff neurologist and Director of the MG Clinic in London, Ontario, the majority of Dr. Nicolle's clinical practice is devoted to the diagnosis and management of patients with myasthenia gravis. He currently holds the position of an Associate Professor in Neurology at the University of Western Ontario, London, Ontario, Canada, and is Director of the MG Clinic and the EMG Laboratory at the London Health Sciences Centre. He has published many articles on MG, its diagnosis and treatment, and is involved with ongoing research projects in MG and its electrodiagnosis.